NEUROTOXICITY GUIDEBOOK

NEUROTOXICITY GUIDEBOOK

Raymond Singer

VNR | VAN NOSTRAND REINHOLD
New York

Copyright © 1990 by Van Nostrand Reinhold

Library of Congress Catalog Card Number 90-33678

ISBN 0-442-23530-5

Manufactured in the United States of America

Published by Van Nostrand Reinhold
115 Fifth Avenue
New York, New York 10003

Chapman and Hall
2-6 Boundary Row
London, SE 1 8HN

Thomas Nelson Australia
102 Dodds Street
South Melbourne 3205
Victoria, Australia

Nelson Canada
1120 Birchmount Road
Scarborough, Ontario M1K 5G4, Canada

16 15 14 13 12 11 10 9 8 7 6 5 4 3 2 1

Library of Congress Cataloging-in-Publication Data

Singer, Raymond M.
   Neurotoxicology guidebook/Raymond M. Singer.
      p.   cm.
   Includes bibliographical references.
   ISBN 0-442-23530-5
   1. Neurotoxicology.   I. Title
RC347.5.S57 1990
616.8—dc20   90-33678
                                                  CIP

CONTENTS

FOREWORD, by Philip J. Landrigan, M. D., M. Sc. / ix
PREFACE / xi

1. THE SCOPE OF NEUROTOXICITY / 1

General Overview / 1
Symptoms of Neurotoxicity / 3
Classes of Neurotoxic Chemicals / 8
Types of Consumer Exposure to Neurotoxic Chemicals / 15
Ramifications of Neurotoxicity / 24
Costs of Neurotoxicity / 30
Regulation of Neurotoxicity / 33
References / 36

2. EVALUATION OF NEUROTOXICITY / 40

Introduction / 40
Biological Monitoring / 41
Monitoring Nervous System Function / 45
Description of the Neurotoxicity Screening Survey / 46
Psychometric Testing / 51
Neurophysiological Tests / 55
References / 60

3. MODEL NEUROTOXICITY SCREENING PROGRAM / 64

Overview of Neurotoxicity Prevention Programs / 64
Purposes of the Neurotoxicity Screening Program / 65
Applications of Neurotoxicity Screening Programs / 65
Design of a Model Neurotoxicity Screening Program / 65
Statistical Aspects of Neurotoxicity Screening Programs / 66
Modules of Neurotoxicity Screening Programs / 67
Data Analysis / 75
Followup / 76
References / 77

4. FORENSIC ASPECTS OF NEUROTOXICITY / 80

Corporate and Managerial Reasons for Concerns about Neurotoxicity /
80
Civil Suits / 81
Worker's Compensation / 87
Criminal Liability for Toxic Injury / 87
Is Ignorance Bliss? / 89
Forensic Evaluation of Single Cases of Neurotoxicity / 91
References / 91

5. SELECTED NEUROTOXICITY CASE REPORTS / 94

Forensic Neurotoxicologic Report of Michael Small / 94
Forensic Neurotoxicologic Report of John Benson / 99
Forensic Neurotoxicologic Report of John Strong / 109
Forensic Neurotoxicologic Report of Billy Thompson / 114
Neurotoxicity Evaluation of Gregory Depark / 122
Neurotoxicologic and Neuropsychologic Evaluation of Kenneth
Deforest / 127
Appendix—Neurotoxicity of Hydrogen Sulfide / 131
References / 131
Formaldehyde Case Report 1—Urea Formaldehyde Foam Insulation
Exposure of Ellen White / 132
Case Reports of Urea Formaldehyde Foam Insulation Exposure of a
Family—
Case 1: Tony Verde / 139
Case 2: Linda Verde / 143
Appendix—Technical Factors of UFFI Installation / 147
References / 148

6. NEUROTOXICITY OF SELECTED SUBSTANCES / 149

The Neurotoxicity of Ammonia / 149
References / 151
Acute Toxicity and Chronic Toxicity of Benzene / 152
References / 154
Acute Toxicity and Chronic Toxicity of Toluene / 154
References / 157
Carbon Monoxide Toxicity / 158
References / 160
The Toxicity of Chlordane and Heptachlor / 160
References / 165

Formaldehyde Neurotoxicity / 166
References / 174
Appendix—Pressed Wood Products / 176
Gasoline Toxicity / 178
Organic Lead / 180
Cadmium / 181
Manganese / 182
References / 183
Organic Mercury Toxicity / 184
References / 187
Organophosphate Neurotoxicity / 188
Appendix—Thimet / 192
References / 192
Polychlorinated Biphenyls (PCBs) / 193
References / 199
Radiation Neurotoxicity / 200
Appendix—Glial Cells / 206
References / 206

INDEX / 209

FOREWORD

Neurologic injury caused by toxic chemicals in the environment is an important, but insufficiently studied and poorly defined problem in public health.

The recognition that environmental chemicals may cause neurological injury first arose from the study of cases of acute illness in persons exposed to toxins at high dose rates, cases of encephalopathy in children who had ingested chips of lead-based paint, and organophosphorus poisoning following exposure to pesticides. That recognition was substantially confirmed by the discovery that environmental toxins had been responsible for major epidemics of neurological impairment. These epidemics included blindness and ataxia caused by ingestion of organic mercury in Minimata Bay, Japan and in Iraq; spinal cord degeneration and peripheral neuropathy caused by tri-orthocresyl phosphate (TOCP) in cooking oil in Morocco and in bootleg liquor in the United States; ataxia, dementia, and peripheral neuropathy caused by the pesticide kepone in Hopewell, Virginia; and epidemic parkinsonism caused by MPTP, a contaminant of synthetic heroin, in California and Hawaii. These epidemics affected thousands of people, and they established clearly that toxic chemicals in the environment can cause neurological illness. However, a major question left unanswered by the study of these epidemics is whether the observed causal associations were isolated events, or whether they were examples of a widespread and pervasive association between toxic environmental chemicals and neurological impairment. This is one of the central questions which this volume addresses.

The discovery in recent years of subclinical neurotoxicity adds yet another dimension to the consideration of environmental neurotoxicology. "Subclinical toxicity" refers to the concept that toxic chemicals, neurotoxins among them, can cause toxic effects at levels of exposure too low to produce signs and symptoms that are evident in the standard medical evaluation. These changes may include loss of intelligence, alteration of behavior, impairment in reasoning ability, shortening of attention span, and fatigue. Environmental chemicals that have been shown capable of causing subclinical neurotoxicity include lead, organophosphate pesticides, certain chlorinated hydrocarbons, organic solvents, and mercury; these are compounds to which several million Americans are exposed regularly at work, and to which tens of millions or more are exposed in the general environment. Although subtle in their presentation, the changes in neurological function produced by subclinical neurotoxicity may be devastating in their effect. Moreover, because the central nervous system has little capacity for repair, the alterations of subclinical neurotoxicity are usually irreversible.

The discovery of subclinical neurotoxicity raises the disturbing possibility that some undefined fraction of chronic neurologic illness in the American population—including such diseases as dementia, parkinsonism, motor neuron disease, and demyelinating illness—may be caused by chronic, low-level exposure to environmental neurotoxins.

A major need in environmental neurotoxicity is to develop biological markers which will permit early documentation of exposure to neurotoxins, and early diagnosis of neurological impairment at a stage when the progress of the illness may still be halted, and when the occurrence of additional cases in others members of an exposed population can potentially be prevented.

The major contribution of this volume is to outline an approach to the development of functional biological markers of neurotoxicity. The volume considers types of exposure to neurotoxic chemicals, the ramifications of neurotoxicity, the development of test batteries, and finally it outlines a model neurotoxicity testing program.

The information presented in this volume should be of great interest both to the specialist and to the practitioner in the rapidly evolving field of environmental neurotoxicity.

Philip J. Landrigan, M.D., M.Sc.

PREFACE

This book was written to inform the educated public about the potential hazards of neurotoxic substances. The impetus for this book was a telephone call in June, 1988, from Mr. Robert Esposito of Van Nostrand Reinhold. He wanted to know if I would be willing to write a book on neurotoxicity that would be suitable for industrial hygienists, safety professionals, occupational health personnel, and others interested in neurotoxicity, including psychologists, neuropsychologists, physicians, risk analyzers, and government regulators.

I felt that there was indeed a pressing need for such a text. During my postdoctoral studies of environmental sciences, I became aware that people were being exposed to neurotoxic substances in the workplace without proper monitoring for possible illness. I was also concerned that neurotoxic substances were widely disseminated in our immediate and global environment, with very little public awareness of the actual toxicity that could result. I agreed to write *Neurotoxicity Guidebook*, and hope that readers will be moved to respond appropriately to the warnings it contains.

ACKNOWLEDGMENTS

Dr. José Valciukas, a pioneer of human neurotoxicology, was instrumental in the development of my skills and knowledge of neurotoxicology. I gratefully acknowledge his help and support over the past 10 years.

Dr. Ruth Lilis and Dr. William Nicholson have generously shared their expertise with me during my formative years as a post-doctoral student of Environmental Epidemiology at Mt. Sinai School of Medicine. Their contributions to occupational and environmental medicine are important and enduring.

Dr. Irving Selikoff has been an inspiration to me and a generation of scientists and doctors dedicated to improving public health. In addition to being a prescient and sensitive scientist, Dr. Selikoff is a gifted speaker. With majestic words and bearing, Dr. Selikoff is able to encourage and guide his listeners to serve humanity with diligence and compassion.

Dr. Selikoff's pioneering work in the study of asbestos hazards has been widely recognized. He brought the world's attention to this subject. In large part through the efforts of Dr. Selikoff, the hazards of asbestos have now become well known.

Dr. Selikoff has led us to examine the subtle yet potentially devastating effects of low-level exposures to toxic substances. He expounded a major paradigm of toxicology: that low-level, long-term toxicity can cause illness years after exposure, even if symptoms are not immediately apparent. This paradigm is especially relevant to neurotoxicology.

Through hard work, dedication and competence, Dr. Selikoff established the Environmental Sciences Laboratory at the Mt. Sinai School of Medicine. This laboratory supported countless studies of occupational and environmental health, and nurtured many clinicians and researchers who have performed important work in their fields.

Dr. Selikoff's contributions to public health touch everyone in the modern world. The impact and reach of his work deserves the highest accolades of medical science.

* * *

Special thanks are extended to my wife, Wendy, for her boundless love and generosity; and to our children, Asher and Eva, who cheer and inspire me everyday.

1

THE SCOPE OF NEUROTOXICITY

GENERAL OVERVIEW

A neurotoxic substance is a substance that is harmful or poisonous to the nervous system. The condition that arises from exposure to the substance is called neurotoxicity.

Perhaps the most well known neurotoxic substance is lead. Lead poisoning can cause brain damage, mental retardation, and personality changes such as irritability. The downfall of the Roman Empire has been attributed to lead poisoning from many sources: lead in the water supply attributable to lead plumbing; possible food contamination from lead plates; and contamination from vessels used for preparing or storing wine (Weeden, 1984). Lead was also added to wine and other foods as a preservative and sweetener (Smith, 1986). Modern neurotoxicologists have wondered if the well-documented cruelty of the Roman aristocracy was due in part to irritability and other nervous system dysfunction from lead poisoning.

The phrase ''mad as a hatter'' is thought to refer to the peculiar behavior of hat makers who used mercury to process pelt into felt. Mercury is a well-known neurotoxic agent which has been linked with several types of mental disturbance. A few years ago, I examined a mercury-exposed worker who indeed exhibited the quirky, flighty behavior of the ''mad hatter'' as depicted in Lewis Carroll's *Alice in Wonderland*. The worker had a reputation among his co-workers as being unpredictable and odd.

Even Sir Isaac Newton is thought to have suffered from mercury poisoning. Newton appeared to be mentally ill around 1692, at which time he was using mercury in his alchemy experiments. Although some historians have attributed his odd behavior to overwork or to other causes of stress, high levels of mercury were found in Newton's hair during recent chemical tests. The levels were 197 ppm, compared with the ''normal'' value of 5.1 ppm. Although Newton appears to have eventually stopped his mercury experiments, his scientific achievements were never again equal to those of his pre-alchemical years (Broad, 1981).

Until recently, the octane level of most gasoline sold in the United States was raised by gasoline blenders who added organic lead compounds. These organic lead compounds are much more neurotoxic than is inorganic lead, and these compounds have been found in the nervous system of the general urban population of the United States when autopsies were performed (Bondy, 1988). Although many people are aware that children are particularly sensitive to the toxic effects of lead, adults are also affected (Valciukas et al, 1985; Singer et al., 1983).

Unusual sources of lead poisoning are occasionally found. For example, in the Middle East, lead contamination has resulted from a process used to grind flour for pita bread. On occasion (or possibly frequently), the devices used to grind wheat into flour for pita bread are manufactured with lead, which eventually contaminates the flour and bread. The flour is ground by a stone wheel, connected to an axle by a bar made from lead, and the lead dust falls into the flour (Hershko, 1984).

Organophosphate pesticides were developed as nerve gases (e.g., Tabun and Sarin) during World War II (Ecobichon and Joy, 1982). After the war, organophosphates were commercially produced as insecticides. It is ironic that the organophosphates, which are now widely used because they rapidly kill unwanted insects, were first developed for their similar effect on humans.

The organochlorine pesticides persist in the environment. This persistence was considered beneficial as it reduced the number of times that the pesticides had to be applied. The Nobel Prize in Medicine in 1948 was awarded to the inventor of DDT (Ecobichon and Joy, 1982). Since that time, DDT has been found to have a number of negative side effects, including the ability to accumulate in animal and human fat. DDT has been banned in the U.S. because 1) it causes health problems in wildlife due to bio-accumulation as animals feed on lower life forms; and 2) because it causes cancer in animals. Despite the ban, DDT and its metabolites remain in the fat of most of the U.S. population; during the period 1970-1975, almost 100% of human tissue samples had detectible amounts of DDT (Schneider, 1979). In addition, it enters the food supply through imported food (NRDC, 1984).

What will be the effect of various low-level neurotoxic contamination of the human nervous system (lead, DDT, other pesticides in food, air, and water)? How can this effect be quantified, as the exposures are uncontrolled? What effect do these substances have on the mental and emotional health of modern man?

We have no assurance that random and continuous exposure to neurotoxic substances are not impairing our nervous system functions. Evidence mounts that there is no threshold of effect for neurotoxic substances such as lead. Logically speaking, biological organisms such as man do not have an unlimited capacity to withstand toxic insults; the organism can be overloaded by multiple, low-level exposure to toxic substances. Considering the effects of many of the other neurotoxic substances to which we are exposed, the situation can be seen to pose an important public health dilemma.

Workers who have been exposed to neurotoxic substances are at special risk of developing neurotoxicity. They should be carefully monitored for the "early warning signs" of neurotoxicity so that permanent nervous system damage can be averted or minimized.

SYMPTOMS OF NEUROTOXICITY

Descriptions of the symptoms of neurotoxicity can be found in Anger and Johnson (1985). In practice, the symptoms of chronic neurotoxicity caused by the various substances are similar. They include:

1. Personality changes
   a. Irritability
   b. Social withdrawal
   c. Amotivation (disturbance of executive function)
2. Mental changes
   a. Problems with memory for recent events
   b. Concentration difficulties
   c. Mental slowness
3. Sleep disturbance
4. Chronic fatigue
5. Headache
6. Sexual dysfunction
7. Numbness in the hands or feet (depends upon the substance)
8. Recognition that there has been a loss of mental function

Additional symptoms are motor incoordination, sensory disturbances, and psychosis.

The symptoms of neurotoxicity have been described in different ways, because of variations in language and in the psychosocial expressions of disease. For example, fatigue has been characterized as neurasthenia, weakness, or depression; irritability has been described as excitability or anxiety; sexual dysfunction has been called loss of libido. Despite the differences in the expression of symptoms and their description, this list of terms captures the essential aspects of the symptoms of neurotoxicity.

Personality Changes

Irritability can be expressed in many different ways. Commonly it is experienced as an increase in arguments with friends, family, and neighbors. There may be problems with the law, such as speeding tickets or public disturbances.

Neurotoxicity reduces mental and emotional abilities, so there will be a reduced ability to perceive, remember, etc., leading in turn to the inability of an individual to express himself or herself and make changes in the social and physical environment. Irritability can result in social withdrawal, as the person finds it increasingly difficult to tolerate the little frustrations that are present in all relationships. The person with neurotoxicity may not be aware he or she has been undergoing decrements in mental and emotional function, and this will increase the level of frustration and irritability.

Social withdrawal occurs as the person with neurotoxicity becomes increasingly frustrated with their functional abilities. The individual may feel that people are staring. This ''paranoia'' may have some basis in fact, as the person may be behaving somewhat peculiarly, and people who interact with the individual may have to pay special attention to determine the nature of their interpersonal communication. As neurotoxicity develops, there will be gaps in the ability to find words, and to understand what others are saying.

Amotivation or disturbances of executive function describes the disorganization of behavior that occurs with brain dysfunction and deterioration. The person with neurotoxicity will have reduced ability to plan, as the thinking processes are disturbed. Abstract thinking becomes impaired, with reduced understanding of the connection between various thoughts, underlying principles, and other cognitive elements. The person appears to be depressed, with psychomotor slowing and feelings of hopelessness.

Mental Changes

Problems with Memory for Recent Events. This symptom will be expressed as forgetfulness, confusion, absent-mindedness, spells, and a reduced responsiveness to the social and physical environment. Long-term memory is often relatively preserved, which may be surprising to the observer. This occurs because neurotoxicity has less effect on memories that have been consolidated within a network of associations to other memories, than on memories that are new.

For investigative purposes, psychologists have divided memory into short-term memory (which includes immediate or eidetic memory and recent memory); delayed memory (memory for events occurring more than 30 minutes ago); and long-term memory. Short-term and delayed memory is affected by neurotoxicity, but long-term memory, that is, memories of events that have been well-learned and mentally rehearsed, particularly if these memories were entered prior to exposure, will remain relatively intact.

Concentration Difficulties. The affected person will find it hard to keep their mind focused. Their thoughts will drift and seem fuzzy. There appears to be a reduction in the ability of the mind to inhibit responses to extraneous stimulation.

One of the primary functions of the mind is to serve as a filtering device. Living organisms are constantly bombarded with all types of stimulation, both internally and externally generated. Our eyes are exposed to light of various colors, arriving in myriad shapes; our eardrums are exposed to sound emanating from many sources. Such descriptions could be composed for all the senses. Along with sensory input, there are cognitive inputs in the form of thoughts, images, fantasies, etc. In order to function effectively, the mind must automatically screen the salient from the less salient sources of mental input. If this function is impaired, a person will appear to be scatter-brained, flighty, moody, etc.

Mental Slowness. This symptom can be expressed as dullness, confusion, difficulty following a conversation, understanding what is read, or following directions.

Neurotoxic chemicals can interfere with the fatty substance that surrounds the nerve cells, the "white matter." This fatty substance (myelin) acts to electrically insulate an individual nerve from the surrounding nerves, and promotes rapid nerve response. When the myelin is degraded, as can occur with many neurotoxic substances, there will be a reduction in brain and nerve conduction velocity, and the amplitude of nerve responsiveness (evoked potential). This degraded response may be observed as mental slowness.

Sleep Disturbance. Sleep patterns are regulated by the secretion of neurohormones that control the degree of wakefulness. These hormones are normally secreted in rhythms corresponding with periods of light and darkness that form day and night. With diffuse brain dysfunction, such as often occurs when a person is affected by neurotoxic chemicals, the pattern of sleep is disrupted, leading to difficulties in falling asleep or staying asleep. This disturbance creates or contributes to the condition of chronic fatigue that is often seen in neurotoxicity patients. Some will find that they sleep much longer than in the past, while others will find that they sleep for shorter periods than in the past.

Chronic Fatigue. Neurotoxicity patients report that they are constantly tired. They are not able to physically move about as they did in the past, and have reduced ability to lift, carry, climb stairs, walk distances, or stay awake. This will be a main factor in their reduced ability to work.

When the brain is functioning less efficiently, activities will take more effort. Memory lapses result in extra, unnecessary activity in attempts to maintain the quality and quantity of activity that occurred prior to the illness. Lack of motor coordination results in easily fatigued muscles. The brain itself may require more energy as it attempts to maintain mental and emotional function. Emotional disturbance resulting from brain dysfunction creates stress which is tiring.

Fatigue can result from dysfunction of the autonomic nervous system. This system controls the heart, digestion, elimination, etc. When diffuse brain dysfunction occurs, the nervous system has less ability to control bodily functions. In turn, as body systems cease to operate properly, an additional negative effect on other organs will occur. As organ function is reduced, any activity becomes more tiring, hence the symptom of fatigue.

When a patient presents these symptoms of chronic fatigue, a doctor may diagnose the illness as depression. Depression can result from the loss of previous levels of ability. Sometimes doctors examine a depressed patient without considering neurotoxicity as a factor and think that the depression can be treated with drugs or therapy. Because a patient appears to have some of the symptoms of clinical depression (i.e., fatigue) a physician may prescribe anti-depressant medication. These drugs may help some patients initially, but their use may mask the cause of the condition and therefore lead to further deterioration. Neurologically active medication (tranquilizers, etc.) may also pose their own risk of brain damage with continued use.

Patients with neurotoxicity often do not have the hallmark symptoms of depression, such as suicidal thoughts or actions, feelings of low self worth and low self esteem, except as secondary symptoms to physical and mental illness caused by chemical toxicity. When faced with a patient who shows symptoms reminiscent of neurotoxicity, it is important to explore neurotoxic exposures as a possible cause of the symptoms.

Headache.   The brain has no pain receptors. This is one reason why neurotoxic chemicals are particularly hazardous. Humans have no direct perception that brain cells are being destroyed or weakened. Pain provides an early warning system of impending injury and disease, and therefore serves an important protective function for our survival. The brain is not provided with such a mechanism.

Headache is thought to originate from the blood vessels or the coverings of the brain (meninges). Muscle contraction headache, also termed tension headache, is described as a pain that is dull, tight, pressing, and constant, and occurs on both sides of the head. Notwithstanding the nomenclature, the cause is unknown, and it may not involve muscle contraction. A current hypothesis states that the pain is due to a depletion of amines or brain chemicals in the pain control system of the brain (Rose, 1987).

Migraine headaches are often diagnosed when the pain is on one side of the head, is severe and incapacitating, is preceded by some type of warning or characteristic sensations (called an aura), and is accompanied by gastrointestinal upset.

Combined, mixed or tension-vascular headaches, are diagnosed when symptoms do not fall nearly within one diagnostic category. However, some researchers believe that all headaches fall within one continuous clinical spectrum, varying in severity rather than in type.

Headache can result from increased pressure on sensitive cranial tissue (cranial vault) due to injury to brain tissue. Such injury can result in swelling and watery secretions.

Whatever the cause may be, neurotoxicity often results in chronic headaches. For neurotoxic diagnostic purposes, further classification or determination of cause may not be necessary.

Sexual Dysfunction.   The type of dysfunction seen in males affected by neurotoxicity is difficulty in maintaining an erection. In both sexes there may be reduced desire for sexual relations, perhaps secondary to fatigue and irritability. These difficulties may have a unified origin within the neurohormonal system.

Due to the shame associated with sexual dysfunction, this symptom is often not discussed by a person affected by neurotoxicity. Although it is shameful and embarrassing not to be able to think clearly, the shame of impaired ''manhood'' seems to be greater. This symptom may therefore not be reported in research literature or clinical records, while it may well be present.

Numbness in the Hands or Feet.   Under conditions of chronic low-level exposure to substances, a neurotoxic agent may damage the peripheral nerves. Because the nerves that serve the feet and hands have very long axons, the source of nerve vitality tends to be located far from the nerve endings, resulting in greater susceptibility to disruption of nerve nutrition and maintenance. Neurotoxicity results in symptoms affecting the arms and perhaps more frequently, the legs and feet. Disruption of the peripheral nervous system may be described by the patient as numbness, tingling, ''pins and needles'' sensation, or a feeling that the limb ''falls asleep''.

Recognition That There Has Been a Loss of Mental Function.   This symptom is most apparent following acute injury by neurotoxic substances. The person will remember that at one time they functioned more effectively, both mentally and interpersonally. They can well recall memories of their lives prior to the exposure, because of the retention of long-term memory, and they can contrast past intact cognitive and emotional function with current function. For example, family relations often sour after neurotoxicity occurs, yet the person affected can remember when family life was satisfactory. The person may have been an avid reader, yet now cannot read due to visual perception defects or impairment of the ability to concentrate when reading.

This symptom as a rule does not occur during the early stages of chronic neurotoxicity, as mental impairment may be subtle. The person may have a dim awareness that something is wrong with their mental and emotional capacities, yet be unable to pinpoint the source of the discomfort.

The previously described symptom occur frequently with neurotoxicity. The following symptoms can develop as the condition worsens.

Motor Incoordination. This symptom can be seen as difficulty in walking, reduced manual dexterity, the dropping of tools, and can progress to motor loss. Neurotoxicity may be misdiagnosed as multiple sclerosis; "MS-like" disease; amyotrophic lateral sclerosis; opsoclonos-myoclonos; seizures; and other diseases affecting the neuromotor system (Singer, 1990).

Sensory Disturbances. Blindness, hearing loss, pain, burning sensations, and kinesthetic dysfunction are examples of sensory disturbance that can occur as neurotoxicity progresses. As the peripheral and central nervous system degenerates, the nerves begin misfiring and transmitting false or inaccurate information to the central nervous system. Any sensory system can be affected, to the point of system failure.

Psychosis. To the psychologist, this is perhaps the most pathetic outcome of neurotoxicity. Patients with this condition may be diagnosed as schizophrenic, schizoid, paranoid, and psychotic. They develop hallucinations, impaired ability to communicate, and impaired ability to function in society. (For descriptions of such cases, see Singer, 1987b, and Chapter 5.)

CLASSES OF NEUROTOXIC CHEMICALS

Solvents, pesticides, herbicides and heavy metals are among the many substances which are toxic to the nervous system. The majority of industrial workers who work with hazardous chemicals are probably exposed to neurotoxic chemicals.

It is impossible to cite all the manufactured products that are neurotoxic, because of the rapid proliferation of new synthesized products, and the lack of pre-market neurotoxicologic testing. In 1976, it was estimated that more than 1,000 new compounds were being developed each year and added to the approximately 40,000 chemicals and 2,000,000 mixtures already in industrial use

(EPA, 1976). Most commercial substances have not even been examined for neurotoxicity (Williams et al., 1987). As of 1989, thorough neurotoxicity testing of commercial products is not practiced.

According to the World Health Organization (WHO, 1986), since the 1970s, ". . . it has become evident that low-level exposure to certain toxic agents can produce deleterious effects that may be discovered only when appropriate procedures are used. While there are still episodes of large scale poisonings, concern has shifted to the more subtle deficits that reduce functioning of the nervous system in less obvious, but still important ways, so that intelligence, memory, emotion, and other complex neural functions are affected . . .

". . . [I]t is not known how often insidious problems of neurotoxicity may lie undetected because effects are incorrectly attributed to other conditions (e.g., advancing age, mood disorders) or misdiagnosed. The early and incipient stages of intoxications produced by environmental agents are frequently marked by vagueness and ambiguity . . . thus the potential is large for the occurrence of subtle, undetected effects, which nonetheless have an important bearing on the quality of life."

Landrigan et al. (1980) reviewed three epidemics of occupational neurotoxicity that had been detected, almost randomly, before 1980. The authors emphasized that the discovered outbreaks underscore the vulnerability of chemical workers to neurotoxins. They hypothesized that large, more easily recognized epidemics of neurotoxic illness represent the easily visible extreme of a larger, more diffuse problem. The authors thought that many more small clusters and single cases of neurologic disease may be caused by occupational exposure to toxic chemicals.

More than 850 chemicals have been identified as producers of neurobehavioral disorders (Anger and Johnson, 1985). Most of these chemicals fall into the categories of solvents, pesticides and metals.

Table 1-1 shows the chemicals (approximately 200) for which workplace regulations were set, in part because of neurotoxicity. Regulations underestimate the risk from neurotoxic chemicals, as the effects of chronic exposure to low-levels of neurotoxicants are often unrecognized. Table 1-2 shows the chemical groupings in which 10 or more neurotoxic chemicals are found. Table 1-3 shows common neurotoxic chemicals which are recognized by the US Center for Disease Control.

From a different perspective, Table 1-4 shows a list of methemoglobin formers, a factor that can induce brain neurotoxicity. Table 1-5 shows a list of asphyxiants, which can produce brain neurotoxicity. Table 1-6 shows a list of central nervous system depressants; Table 1-7 shows neurotoxic agents that produce convulsions.

Table 1-1. Chemicals for which ACGIH TLVs were set in part because of neurotoxicity.

Abate® (Temephos)
Acetonitrille (methyl cyanide)
Acrylamide
Aldrin
Allyl alcohol
Anisidine
Barium
Baygon® (Propoxur)
Benzyl chloride
Bromine pentafloride
n-Butyl alcohol
sec-Butyl alcohol
tert-Butyl alcohol
p-t-Butyltoluene Camphor
Camphor
Carbaryl
Carbon disulfide
Carbon tetrachloride
Chlordane
Chlorinated camphene 60% (Toxaphene)
Chlorine trifluoride
Chlorobenzene
Chlorobromomethane
Chloropyrifos (Dursban)
Cobalt hydrocarbonyl
Cumene
Cyanides
Cyclohexylamnine
Cyclopentadiene
Cyclopentane
Decaborane
Demeton
Diazinon
Diborane
Dibrom®
Dibutyl phosphate
Dichloroacetylene
p-Dichlorobenzene
Dichlorodiphenyltrichloroethane (DDT)
2,4-Dichlorophenoxyacetic acid (2,4-D)
Dichloroterafluoro-ethane (Freon 114)
Dichlorvos (DDVP)
Dicrotophos
Dieldrin
Diethanolamine
Diethylamine
Diethyl ketone
Difluordibromomethane (Freon 12B2)
Diisopropylamine
Dimethylanaline
1,1-Dimethylhydrazine

Dioxathion
Dipropylene glycol methyl ether (DPGME)
Diquat
Disulfoton
Dyfonate
EPN
Ethanolamine
Ethion
Ethyl amyl ketone
Ethyl bromide
Ethyl butyl ketone
Ethyl ether (diethyl ether)
Ethyl mercaptan
Ethylene chlorohydrin
Ethylene glycol dinitrate
N-Ethylmorpholine
Fenamiphos
Fensulfothion
Fenthion
Halothane
n-Heptane
Hexachlorocyclo-pentadiene
Hexachloroethane
n-Hexane
Hydrogen cyanide
Hydrogen selenide
Hydrogen sulfide
Hydroquione
Iron pentacarbonyl
Isoamyl alcohol
Isophorone
N-Isopropylaniline
Isopropyl ether
Lead, inorganic
Lindane
Manganese (and compounds)
Manganese cyclopentadienyl tricarbonyl (MCT)
Manganese tetroxide
Mercury, alkyl
Mercury, not alkyl
Mesityl oxide
Methomyl
4-Methoxyphenol
Methyl acetate
Methyl alcohol (Methanol)
Methyl bromide (monobromomethane)
Methyl-n-butyl ketone (MBK)
Methyl chloride (monochloromethane)
Methyl chloroform
Methyl demeton
Methylene chloride

10

Table 1-1. (*Continued*)

Methyl ethyl ketone (MEK; 2- Butanone)
Methyl mercaptan
Methyl parathion
Methyl propyl ketone
Methyl silicate
Methylacrylonitrille
Methylcyclohexane
o-Methylcyclohexanone
2-Methylcyclopentanedienyl manganese
   tricarbonyl (CI-2)
Metrizabin
Monocrotophos
Morpholine
Naphthalene
Naptha
Nickel carbonyl
Nitromethane
2-Nitropropane
Osmium tetroxide
Parathion
Pentaborane
Pentane
Perchloroethylene (tetrachloroethylene)
Phenyl ether
Phenyl mercaptan
Phenylphosphine
Phorate
Phosdrin (Mevinphos)
Phosphorus oxychloride
1 Propanol (n-propyl alcohol)
Propargyl alcohol
1,2-Propylene glycol dinitrate
Propylene glycol monoethyl ether
Propylene oxide

Pyridine
Quinone
Ronnel
Selenium (and compounds)
Selenium hexafluoride
Stoddard solvent (mineral spirits; white spirits)
Strychnine
Sulfuryl fluoride
Sulprofos
Tellurium
1,1,2,2-tetra-chloroethane (acetylene
   tetrachloride)
Tetraethyl dithionopyrophosphate (TEDP)
Tetraethyl lead (TEL)
Tetraethyl pyrophosphate (TEPP)
Tetrahydrofuran (THF)
Tetramethyl lead (TML)
Tetramethyl succinonitrille (TMSN)
Tetranitromethane
Tetryl
Thallium
Tin, organic
Toulene
Tributyl phosphate
Trichloracetic acid
1,1,2-Trichloethane (vinyl trichloride)
Trichloroethylene
Trichlohexyltin hydrochloride
Trimethyl benzene
Trimethyl phosphite
Triorthocresyl phosphate (TOCP)
Tripheny phosphate (TPP)
Xylene

Source: Adapted from Anger, 1984.

Table 1-2. Chemical groupings in which ten or more neurotoxic chemicals are found.

Alcohols
Alicyclic hydrocarbons
Aliphatic and alicyclic amines
Aliphatic carboxyl acids
Aliphatic hydrocarbons
Aliphatic nitro compounds,
   nitrates, and nitrites
Aromatic hydrocarbons
Cyanides and nitriles
Esters of aromatic monocarboxylic acids
   and monoalcohols
Ethers

Glycol derivatives
Halogenated aliphatic hydrocarbons containing
   Cl, Br, and I
Halogenated cyclic hydrocarbons
Ketones
Metals
Nitrogen compounds
Organic phosphates
Organic phosphorous esters
Organic sulfur compounds
Phenols and phenolic compound

Source: Anger 1986. *Patty's Industrial Hygiene and Toxicology*, Vol. 2, New York: John Wiley & Sons. 1981–1982.

Table 1-3. Commonly used industrial chemicals recognized as neurotoxic.

Acetyl ethyl tetramethyl tetralin	Hydroquinone
Acetyl pyridine	Lead
Acrylamide	Lead, tetraethyl
Adiponitrile	Letophos
Alkyl phosphates	Malonitrile
Aluminum	Manganese
Aniline	Mercury
Arsenic, inorganic	Methanol
Arsine	Methyl bromide
Aryl phosphates	Methyl n-butyl ketone
Azide	Methyl chloride
Barium	Nickel (carbonyl)
Benzene	Nitrogen trichloride
Boron	Organochlorine insecticides
p-Bromophenyl acetylurea	Organophosphate esters
Cadmium	Organotins (triethytin)
Carbon disulfide	Paraquat
Carbon monoxide	Phenol
Carbon tetrachloride	Phenyl mercury
Chlordane	Phthalate esters
Chlordecone	Polybrominated biphenyls (PBBs)
Chloroprene	Selenium
Cobalt	Styrene
Cuprozone	Sulfur dioxide
Cyanide	Tetrachlorobiphenyl
Dichlorodiphenyl trichloroethane (DDT)	Thallium
2,4-Dichlorophenoxy acetic acid (2,4-D)	Toulene
Diethyl ether	Trichloroethylane
Diisopropyl fluorophosphate (DFP)	Triorthocresylphosphate (TDCP)
Dimethyl sulphate	Vanadium, inorganic salt
Ethylene dichloride	Zinc
n-Hexane	Zinc pyridinethione
Hexachlorophene	

Source: CDC, 1986.

Table 1-4. Methemoglobin formers.

Aniline	p-Nitrochlorobenzene
Anisidine, ortho- and para-isomers	Nitrogen trifluoride
Dimethylaniline	Nitrotoluene
Dinitrobenzene, all isomers	Perchloryl fluoride
Dinitrotoluene	n-Propyl nitride
Monomethylaniline	Tetranitromethane
p-Nitroaniline	o-Toluidine
Nitrobenzene	Xylidine
o-Nitrochlorobenzene	

Source: Proctor et al. 1988.

Table 1-5. Asphyxiants.

CHEMICAL ASPHYXIANTS

Acetonitrile	Cyanide (alkali)
Acrylonitrile	Hydrogen cyanide
Carbon monoxide	

SIMPLE ASPHYXIANTS

Acetylene	Hydrogen
Argon, neon and helium	Liquid petroleum gas
Carbon dioxide	Methane
Dichloromonofluoromethane	Nitrogen
Dichlorotetrafluoroethane	Propane
Ethane	Propylene
Ethylene	

Source: Proctor et al. 1988.

Table 1-6. Central nervous system depressants.

Acetaldehyde	Diacetone alcohol
Acetone	Dichlorodifluoromethane
Acetylene dichloride	Dichlorethyl ether
Acrylamide	Difluorodibromomethane
Allyl glycidyl ether	Diglycidyl ether
n-Amyl acetate	Diisobutyl ketone
sec-Amyl acetate	Dipropylene glycol methyl ether
Benzene	2-Ethoxyethyl acetate
Bromoform	Ethyl acetate
1,3-Butadiene	Ethyl alcohol
n-Butyl acetate	Ethyl amyl ketone
sec-Butyl acetate	Ethylbenzene
tert-Butyl acetate	Ethyl bromide
n-Butyl alcohol	Ethyl butyl ketone
sec-Butyl alcohol	Ethyl chloride
tert-Butyl alcohol	Ethylene dibromide
n-Butyl glycidyl ether	Ethylene dichloride
Butyl mercaptan	Ethylene oxide
Carbon disulfide	Ethyl ether
Carbon tetrachloride	Ethyl formate
Chlorobenzene	Ethyl mercaptan
Chlorobromomethane	Ethylidene chloride
Chloroform	Furfuryl alcohol
Cresol, all isomers	Glycidol
Cumene	n-Heptane
Cyclohexane	Hexachloroethane
Cyclohexanol	n-Hexane
Cyclohexanone	sec-Hexyl acetate
Cyclohexene	Isoamyl acetate
Decaborane	Isoamyl alcohol

Table 1-6. (*Continued*)

Isobutyl acetate	Octane
Isobutyl alcohol	Pentaborane
Isopropyl acetate	Pentane
Isopropyl alcohol	Phenyl glycidyl ether
Isopropyl ether	Propyl acetate
Mesityl oxide	*n*-Propyl alcohol
Methyl acetate	Propylene dichloride
Methyl acetylene	Propylene oxide
Methyl acetylene, propadiene mixture	Pyridine
Methylal	Stoddard solvent
Methyl amyl ketone	Styrene
Methyl butyl ketone	Sulfuryl fluoride
Methyl cellosolve acetate	1,1,1,2-Tetrachloro-2,2-difluoroethane
Methylcyclohexane	1,1,2,2-Tetrachloro-1,2-difluoroethane
Methylcyclohexanol	Tetrachloroethane
o-Methylcyclohexanone	Tetrachloroethylene
Methylene chloride	Tetrahydrofuran
Methyl ethyl ketone	Toluene
Methyl formate	1,1,1-Trichloroethane
Methyl iodide	1,1,2-Trichloroethane
Methyl isobutyl carbinol	Trichlorethylene
Methyl isobutyl ketone	Trichlorofluoromethane
Methyl mercaptan	1,2,3-Trichloropropane
Methyl propyl ketone	1,1,2-Trichloro-1,2,2-trifluoroethane
α-Methyl styrene	Turpentine
Naphtha, coal tar	Vinyltoluene
Naphtha, petroleum distillates	Xylene
Nitroethane	

Source: Proctor et al. 1988.

Table 1-7. Convulsive neurotoxic agents.

Aldrin	Methyl iodide
2-Aminopyridine	Methyl mercaptan
Camphor	Monomethylhydrazine
Chlordane	Nicotine
Crag herbicide	Nitromethane
DDT	Oxalic acid
Decaborane	Pentaborane
2,4-Dichlorophenoxyacetic acid	Phenol
Dieldrin	Rotenone
1,1-Dimethylhydrazine	Sodium fluoroacetate
Endrin	Strychnine
Heptachlor	Tetraethyl lead
Hydrazine	Tetramethyl lead
Lindane	Tetramethylsuccinonitrile
Methoxychlor	Thallium, soluble compounds
Methyl bromide	Toxaphene
Methyl chloride	

Source: Proctor et al. 1988.

As these tables show, neurotoxic chemicals abound in industrial settings. It is impossible at this time to state the number of chemicals that are neurotoxic, but the number is very large. As a general guideline, if a substance falls within a category of known or suspected neurotoxic chemicals, then the substance must be suspected of being neurotoxic before it is declared safe.

For a comprehensive review of the neurotoxic effects of selected chemicals, see Johnson (1987). This review categorized the neurotoxic effects of a number of chemicals, and includes clinical reports, epidemiologic and experimental investigations. The neuropsychological effect of specific chemicals are also covered in Hartman (1988).

The Number of Workers Exposed to Neurotoxic Chemicals. The number of workers exposed to neurotoxic chemicals is difficult to estimate, although probably more than 40 million workers are at risk. Table 1-8 (Hartman, 1988) shows a compilation of the number of workers exposed to various neurotoxic chemicals (reaching about 36 million). Anger (1986) lists 65 neurotoxic chemicals with estimated United States exposure populations over one million (Table 1-9). Approximately one third of the 200 industrial chemicals to which more than one million people in the United States are exposed are neurotoxic (NIOSH, 1977).

Table 1-10 lists some occupations and activities at risk for neurotoxic exposure. Table 1-11 shows other industries in which neurotoxic chemicals are found.

Governmental Recognition of Occupational Neurotoxicity. Neurotoxic disorders are on the US National Institute of Safety and Health (NIOSH) List of Ten Leading Work-Related Diseases and Injuries (CDC, 1986), because of their potential severity and because of the large number of workers at risk.

The American Conference of Governmental Industrial Hygienists has identified neurotoxicity as the basis for recommending threshold limit values for 30% of the toxic chemicals most frequently encountered in industry (Anger, 1984).

TYPES OF CONSUMER EXPOSURE TO NEUROTOXIC CHEMICALS

Practically speaking, all people are exposed to neurotoxic chemicals from commercial products at levels that may cause permanent nervous system dysfunction. Two sources will be discussed: petroleum fuel (gasoline, diesel, etc.) and pesticides.

Table 1-8. Subjects at risk for neurotoxic exposure at the workplace.

Neurotoxic Substance	Estimated Numbers at Risk
Alcohols (industrial)	3,851,000
Aliphatic hydrocarbons	2,776,000
Aromatic hydrocarbons	3,611,000
Cadmium	1,400,000
Carbon disulfide	24,000
Carbon tetrachloride	1,379,00
Dichloromethane	2,175,000
N-hexane	764,000
Lead (In children from inorganic paint exposure)	45,000
Lead acetate	103,000
Lead carbonate	183,000
Lead metallic	1,394,00
Lead naphtenate	1,280,000
Lead oxides	1,300,000
Manganese	41,000
Mercury chloride	51,000
Mercury, metallic	24,000
Mercury, nitrate	10,100
Mercury, organic	280,000
Mercury, sulfide	8,900
Perchoroethylene (tetrachloroethylene)	1,596,000
Pesticides (1979)	1,275,000
Rubber solvents (benzene and lacquer diluent)	600,000
Stryene	329,000
Thallium	853,000
Toluene	4,800,000
Trichoroethylene	3,600,000
Xylene	140,000

Source: Hartman, 1988.

Petroleum Fuels

Until recently, lead was added to gasoline in the United States. While use of this additive is being phased out in the United States, it is still added to gasoline in many other countries. Because of the pioneering research by a number of health professionals (Needleman, Landrigan, etc.), U.S. legislators have become aware of the hazards of lead to children, and by regulation are attempting to greatly reduce the lead content of U.S. petroleum fuels. Recent understanding of lead toxicity suggests that there is no threshold of the effects of lead on

Table 1-9. Neurotoxic chemicals with estimated exposure populations exceeding one million[1]

Acetone (1,000 ppm)	Formaldehyde (3 ppm)
Alcohol	Glycerol
Aliphatic hydrocarbons	Hexane (500 ppm)
Alkanes	Isophorone (25 ppm)
Alkyl styrene polymers	Lead (0.05 mg/m^3)
Ammonia (500 ppm)	Lithium grease
Amyl acetate, N- (100 ppm)	Methanol (200 ppm)
Aniline (5 ppm)	Methyl acetate (200 ppm)
Antimony sulfide (0.5 mg/m^3)	Nitrous oxide
Aromatic hydrocarbons	Oil, fuel no. 1
Asphalt	Oil, lube
Benzene (1 ppm)	Petroleum distillates
Butanol	Pine oil
Butyl acetate (150 ppm)	Polymethacrylate resin
Cadmium oxides (0.1 mg/m^3)	Products of combustion
Carbon disulfide (20 ppm)	Propanol, 1-
Carbon tetrachloride (10 ppm)	Propylene glycol (200 ppm)
Chlorinated hydrocarbons	Shellac
Chlorobenzene (75 ppm)	Sodium chloride
Chromium oxides	Solvent
Cresol (5 ppm)	Tetrachloroethylene (100
Cyclohexanol (50 ppm)	ppm)
Cyclohexanone (50 ppm)	Toluene (200 ppm)
Degreaser	Trichlorobenzene
Diacetone alcohol (50 ppm)	Trichloroethylene
Dichlorobenzene, ortho- (50 ppm)	Trichloroflouromethane
Dichlorotetrafluoroethane (1000 ppm)	Tricresyl phosphate (0.1
Diphenylamine	mg/m^3)
Dyes	Tungsten oxides
Ethanol	Turpentine (100 ppm)
Ethyl acetate (400 ppm)	Vinyl chloride
Ethylene glycol (0.2 ppm)	Xylene (100 ppm)
Food additives	

[1]Adapted from Anger, 1986.
[2]Ceiling exposure values.

human health, and that even small amounts may cause nervous system dysfunction.[1] This can occur in adults as well as in children.

As the gasoline additive lead was phased out, other neurotoxic substances were substituted, including benzene, toluene and xylene. These substances pose a hazard because of the vaporization of unburnt fuel; exhaust of partially burnt

---

1. Landrigan (1988) reviewed the effects of low-level lead exposure. Nine percent of all pre-school children have blood lead levels in the dangerous range (25 μg/dl or more). Landrigan cited a number of studies that showed toxic effects of lead at levels below 25 μg/dl.

Table 1-10.   Occupations and activities at risk for neurotoxic exposure.

Occupations and Activities	Neurotoxic Substance
Agriculture and farm workers	Pesticides, herbicides, insecticides, solvents
Chemical and pharmaceutical workers	Industrial and pharmaceutical substances
Degreasers	Trichloroethylene
Dentists and Dental hygienists	Mercury, anesthetic gases
Dry-cleaners	Perchloroethylene, trichloethylene, other solvents
Electronics workers	Lead, methyl ethyl ketone, methylene chloride, tin, trichloroethylene, glycol ether, xylene, chloroform, freon, arsine
Hospital personnel	Alcohols, anesthetic gases, ethylene oxide (cold sterilization)
Laboratory workers	Solvents, mercury, ethylene oxide
Painters	Lead, toluene, xylene, other solvents
Plastics workers	Formaldehyde, styrene, PVCs
Printers	Lead, methanol, methylene chloride, toluene, trichloroethylene, and other solvents
Rayon workers	Carbon disulfide
Steel workers	Lead, other metals
Transportation workers	Lead (in gasoline), carbon monoxide, solvents
Hobbyists	Lead, toluene, glues, solvents

Source: Hartman, 1988.

Table 1-11.   SIC classifications and industries in which neurotoxic chemicals are found.

07 Agricultural services and hunting	34 Fabricated metal products
13 Oil and gas extraction	35 Machinery, except electrical
16 Heavy construction	36 Electrical equipment and supplies
17 Special trade contractors	37 Transportation equipment
19 Ordinance and accessories	38 Instruments and related products
20 Food and kindred products	39 Miscellaneous manufacturing industries
21 Tobacco manufacture	41 Passenger transit
22 Textile mill products	42 Trucking and warehousing
23 Apparel and other textile products	44 Water transportation
24 Lumber and wood products	45 Transportation by air
25 Furniture and fixtures	46 Pipeline transportation
26 Paper and allied products	50 Wholesale trade
27 Printing and publishing	54 Food stores
28 Chemicals and allied products	55 Auto dealers and service stations
29 Petroleum and coal products	58 Eating and drinking places
30 Rubber and plastic products	72 Personal service
31 Leather and leather products	73 Miscellaneous business services
32 Stone, clay and glass products	75 Auto repair, services, and garages
33 Primary metal industries	80 Medical and other health services

Source: Anger, 1986.

fuel; and the creation of benzene and other neurotoxic substances by partial combustion (Singer, 1987a). The neurotoxicity of gasoline and gasoline additives will be reviewed in a later chapter.

The neurotoxicity of gasoline fuel per se, even without additives (see Chapter 6), has escaped the awareness of public regulators of toxic chemicals. Although analysis of this fuel shows a very complex mixture of substances, by itself gasoline is neurotoxic, as are the exhaust fumes. Due to the neurotoxic nature of these substances and the large population that is exposed to these substances, a very large neurotoxic hazard exists.

Although the dimensions of gasoline neurotoxicity remains unexplored, the situation is one of great concern. Until the neurotoxicity of gasoline and related substances has been thoroughly studied, and shown to pose no hazard to the countless people exposed, it seems prudent to recommend gasoline alternatives such as alcohol (ethanol) fuels.

Ethanol provides a much cleaner fuel source with much less chance for neurotoxicity. However, burning ethanol still may contribute to the "greenhouse effect" and possibly to destruction of the ozone layer. Ethanol may be promoted as an interim fuel, until our society develops truly renewable energy sources that are produced and used in a safe and healthy manner—such as solar power.[2]

Pesticides in Food

No one can eat food without pesticides, except for people who grow their own or who have access to naturally grown foods. Unfortunately, there are no studies that demonstrate the safety of human consumption of the multitude of pesticide residue in our daily food, nor are there studies showing that these pesticides in food do not cause permanent, cumulative brain damage.

Modern pesticides were originally developed for warfare. Organophosphates were found to be extremely toxic to humans and therefore efficient for killing animal life in general. The lethality of nerve gases were reduced for commercial use. However, they still maintain their effectiveness in killing species with less capacity of detoxifying their active ingredients. The strength of commercial pesticides is supposedly adjusted so that they do not cause obvious nervous system dysfunction in an exposed population that is active, healthy, and male if the commercial application occurs as directed by the manufacturer, without the usual human error as seen in practice. Unfortunately, pesticides do injure many people. As scientists begin studying people who have been exposed to

---

2. Koshland (1989) states that the development of solar energy technology to supply large amounts of power should be a major priority of our civilization. Fulkerson et al. (1989) estimated that spending of $200 million per year would be sufficient to develop effective solar and other renewable energy sources.

pesticides, they are finding many cases of overt neurotoxicity caused by many types of pesticides. (See the sections on pesticides in Chapter 6.)

Symptoms of pesticide poisoning can be subtle. Mental and emotional dysfunction may develop so gradually that it can go unnoticed for years. As mentioned above, there are no pain cells in the brain to warn of brain cell death or injury. The person affected by neurotoxicity may not know that toxic chemicals can produce neurotoxicity, so awareness of the cause of mental dysfunction will be even less likely. Mental and emotional decrements caused by neurotoxicity are often attributed to "normal aging" by the untrained observer. Neurotoxic effects are cumulative, because brain cells do not regenerate.

Low-level neurotoxicity may go unnoticed because of the following reasons:

1. The effects are subtle.
2. The deterioration is gradual.
3. No pain cells in the brain warn of cell injury.
4. Mental, emotional or nervous dysfunction, if detected, are attributed to "getting old."
5. There is little public awareness that commercial products or toxic chemicals can affect brain function.
6. The person affected is progressively less aware of their situation as neurotoxicity continues, because of the cumulative effect of toxicity.
7. The latency period for senile dementia may be extended, and the appearance of the dementia can occur a long time after exposure.

It seems unlikely that there is a threshold of exposure intensity that must be breached in order for neurotoxicity to occur. A more likely scenario would be injury of cells at low-levels of exposure, with the death of more sensitive nervous tissue at higher exposure levels. Figure 1-1 represents an exposure level in the sublethal range, where the vast number of cells show no injury, a smaller number show some injury, and a few cells die.

There is no evidence that the levels of pesticide residue found in food are harmless. By putting pesticides in the entire food supply, we are conducting a possibly very dangerous experiment.

Pesticides banned for use in the United States can find their way into our food supply via produce from other countries which have less stringent regulations. For example, DDT can still be found in our food supply (NRDC, 1984). In addition to "banned pesticide rebound," third world growers who cannot read the manufacturer's instructions can easily over-apply pesticides. The FDA (GAO, 1989a) is too short-staffed to adequately monitor the pesticide status of imported food. Pesticides which have lost their EPA registration because of toxicity are manufactured in the United States and sent abroad to be used in other countries. Unfortunately for United States citizens, these pesticides return

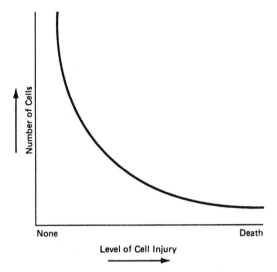

Figure 1-1. Sublethal exposure to a neurotoxic substance.

to the United States on produce and fruit. The EPA does not adequately monitor the export of unregistered pesticides (eg., heptachlor) which are likely to return to the food supply in imported produce. Loopholes in the monitoring system include the following:

1. The EPA allows the export of almost 75% of the unregistered pesticides.
2. The EPA has no system to verify notification by exporting companies.
3. The EPA does not have the authority to prohibit the exporting of pesticides (GAO, 1989b).

A recent study of vegetable samples sold in San Francisco markets found pesticide residue of 19 different pesticides in 44% of the produce (NRDC, 1984). Residues of more than one pesticide (which can lead to synergistic neurotoxicity) were found in 42% of the produce. The most common pesticide found in food was DDT, which had been banned 12 years prior to the study.

The majority of pesticides detected in produce by NRDC (1984) were within the tolerance levels accepted by the EPA. However, tolerances that are acceptable to the U.S. EPA are far from safe. These standards have even been criticized as unsafe by the U. S. General Accounting Office (GAO, 1986a; 1986b).

The EPA's pesticide tolerance levels are unsafe for the following reasons:

1. Neurotoxicity tests are not required, although that is the primary action of most pesticides.

2. Individual sensitivities are not adequately protected (ie., special vulnerability of the old, young, sick, etc.) (Friedman, 1981).
3. The synergistic effects of pesticides are not considered.
4. The cumulative neurotoxic effects of pesticides are not considered.
5. Also not considered is the variable toxicity of pesticides under various exposure conditions, such as circadian rhythm sensitivity, and temperature at the time of exposure.
6. The EPA unrealistically assumes that only small quantities of foods will be eaten, such as less than 7.5 ounces per year of blueberries, melons, radishes, and a long list of other common foods. If a person eats more than 7.5 ounces per year of blueberries, avocados, honeydew melon, etc., they are potentially exposed to more pesticide residue than the EPA considers safe (NRDC, 1984).
7. The EPA relies upon animal studies when setting "acceptable" limits for toxic chemicals. Animal studies, particularly of rodents, when used to evaluate the potential of a substance for human toxicity include the following limitations:
    a. The human nervous system is much more complex than the nervous systems of rodents. Human memory, language, emotions, and other functions can be affected by neurotoxicity in subtle ways that are difficult to detect in rodents.
    b. In the world outside the researcher's laboratory, people are exposed to multiple neurotoxic chemicals simultaneously. This can synergize the effects of one chemical upon another. For example, food may contain multiple pesticides; homes may contain multiple pesticides against cockroaches, termites, etc; dust in air may contain residues of lead from leaded gasoline exhaust dust; and indoor latex paint may contain mercury. Such simultaneous exposure would be difficult to simulate in the laboratory.

All these factors must be considered when the safety of pesticide residue is evaluated.

Pesticides in the Home and Office

A large variety of pesticides are applied to the indoor environment, contributing to indoor air pollution. Chlordane alone has been applied to over 20 million homes in the United States as a termite treatment. Chlordane is very long-acting: it is effective for more than 20 years.

The chlorinated pesticides, of which chlordane is one, were formulated to be both long-lasting and less acutely lethal than the organophosphate pesticides.

An unwanted side-effect of this pesticide design is the risk of both subtle immediate and subtle long-term neurotoxicity.

There are no scientific studies which show the safety of long-term, low level absorption of chlordane or other chlorinated pesticides. Of course, there are no studies of such effects in those who are more susceptible, including children, the elderly, and fetuses. Chlordane will be covered in detail in Chapter 6.

Neurotoxic pesticides are routinely applied in homes, offices, stores, schools, and government buildings. They present an unrecognized and potentially serious hazard to human health.

Herbicides

Herbicides gained notoriety as neurotoxic substances during the Agent Orange litigation. Agent Orange is composed of 2,4,5-trichlorophenoxy acetic acid, 2,4-dichlorophenoxy acetic acid and traces of dioxin. Although dioxin, a by-product of herbicide production, has gained notoriety because of it's extreme toxicity, it is less well known that the herbicides themselves can be neurotoxic (CDC, 1986). Herbicides are routinely applied for lawn maintenance, at locations such as golf courses, playing fields, highways, railroad right-of-ways, and homes. Herbicides are applied to kill dandelions and other broad-leaf plants.

The Agent Orange litigation was the largest personal injury suit in history up to that time, with a settlement value of $180 million. This settlement was based, in part, upon the neurotoxicity of Agent Orange and the findings of neurotoxicity in some of the veterans who were plaintiffs at the test trial.[3]

Formaldehyde

Compared with pesticides, formaldehyde is less toxic, although consumer exposure is extensive. This substance can be found in building insulation (urea foam formaldehyde insulation), particle board, home furnishings and other items. Given a particular set of unfortunate conditions, formaldehyde levels can get high enough to cause permanent nervous system dysfunction and brain damage in susceptible people. Formaldehyde neurotoxicity will be covered in a later chapter.

Waste Products from Manufacturing Concerns

Waste products from manufacturing processes are often more toxic than are the raw materials of manufacture or the finished product. For example, the pro-

---

3. The size of legal settlements in this case may be eclipsed by the reported offer of $470 million dollar settlement of the Bhopal case.

cessing of copper ore results in the release of lead and arsenic with a resulting risk of neurotoxicity (Singer, 1990b). Toxic waste can result from used solvents, which migrate to water supplies. Waste solvents can also be leaked deliberately from transport trucks as they roll down the highway. Other removal tactics include mislabelling and storage on property soon to be abandoned.

Waste disposal sites, both legal and illegal, can pose hazards to workers and community residents. Often we hear of water and air contamination from waste disposal sites. Many types of waste can be present, and neurotoxicity can be suspected with prolonged or sometimes even brief exposure to toxic waste.

The types of neurotoxic waste exposure that I have personally researched include exposures to air which contained solvents that had been used for degreasing of machinery; solvents in drinking water from underground storage tanks; used solvents simply dumped on a property, and which had migrated to the local water supply; and mixed waste from electrical energy generation (coal fired plant) (see Singer, 1987b, for a description of psychosis from toxic waste dump material).

These are just a few sample descriptions of the types of neurotoxic chemicals to which the general U.S. population is exposed.

RAMIFICATIONS OF NEUROTOXICITY

Sensitivity of the Human Nervous System to Toxicity. The human nervous system is the most complex biological organization known to man. There are countless neural connections, perhaps hundreds of endogenous chemicals controlling nervous system function, and long lengths of nervous system tissue. The human nervous system is capable of synthesis and analysis far beyond the abilities of any machines that we have created. It controls all bodily functions, thoughts, the will, desires, communication, etc. On logical grounds alone, the human nervous system would be selected as the human organ most susceptible to disruption from exogenous substances, whether such substances cause subtle deterioration in other organ functions (such as liver detoxification), or whether such substances act directly on nervous system tissue, such as the action of solvents in dissolving the fatty sheaths surrounding many nerves.

Mechanisms of Brain Susceptibility to Toxicity. The human nervous system is extremely sensitive to chemicals. Known neurotransmitters include acetylcholine, dopamine, noradrenaline, GABA, glycine and serotonin (WHO, 1986; Cooper et al., 1986). Neurohormones control brain and other organ functions. Because of the large number of known and potentially unknown endogenous neurochemicals, it may be difficult to predict or specify the neurobehavioral effects of many industrial chemicals as mediated by brain chemicals. The interaction of various toxic substances in the human body may compound the difficulty of predicting neurotoxicity. This topic is explored by Weiss (1986). The general topic of compound effects is discussed by Iyaniwura (1990).

The "blood-brain barrier" (BBB) is the term used to describe a central nervous system (CNS) function of reducing the permeability of brain capillaries to potentially toxic substances in the blood. This selectivity results from several structural and functional differences in brain capillaries relative to those in other tissues (Oldendorf, 1987). Opinions differ on the site of the BBB. Oldendorf believes the BBB to be everywhere, except for a few small regions in the floor of the third ventricle and the area postrema, a small volume of tissue surrounding the caudal extreme of the fourth ventricle; others believe that the BBB excludes the hypothalamic region, the pineal and pituitary glands, and other nervous tissue such as the autonomic ganglia (National Research Council, 1986). Damage to these areas could affect memory, personality, and general vitality. Solutes with a high affinity for membrane lipid relative to water (a high lipid/water partition coefficient) can readily penetrate the BBB. The BBB is not completely impermeable to any plasma solute, although the BBB can slow down the passage of some plasma solutes.

In the presence of almost any lesion which exhibits significant histopathology, regardless of etiology, brain capillary structure changes, and the BBB is lost (Oldendorf, 1987). The BBB does not protect the brain from many types of toxic substances, including lipid soluble substances and gases (including volatile solvents, anesthetic gases, CO_2). Chemicals and drugs, such as mercuric chloride, may increase the permeability of the blood-brain barrier (Katzman, 1981).

Permanency of Neurotoxicity.   Injury to neural tissue disrupts function by destroying cells and interrupting nerve fibers. Because dead nerve cells are not replaced, recovery depends upon regrowth of damaged neuronal branches and the reconnection of the surviving cells. In contrast with the peripheral nervous system, there is little fiber regrowth within the CNS, and many of the functional deficits caused by damage to the brain and spinal cord are permanent (Aguayo, 1987).

Difficulties for Detection of Personal Neurotoxicity.   Mental deterioration from exposure to low-levels of neurotoxic chemicals may not be noticed by the person affected for a number of reasons, including 1) the brain lacks the ability to detect pain resulting from brain cell death or injury, and therefore lacks sensitivity to destruction of brain tissue itself; and 2) mental deterioration often occurs in small increments, so that gradual and subtle change is difficult to notice. Over time such gradual decrements can cause a significant decline in mental function. As a person's mental processes deteriorate, they are less able use to use logic, perception, memory, and other mental processes to determine the extent or cause of mental deterioration.

There is a lack of individual and societal awareness that toxic chemicals can permanently damage brain function, so a person may not look for any cause of functional nervous system decrement. When a person begins having problems with memory or personality, it is unlikely that they or others would even suspect that neurotoxic chemicals may be the cause.

Acute Versus Delayed Neurotoxicity. To the extent there is some awareness of neurotoxicity, the general public may associate neurotoxicity with obvious, acute toxic effects, such as occur after exposure to nerve gas or other high doses of deadly substances. They may not be aware of the subtle effects of neurotoxic chemicals, or the cumulative effects of low-level toxicity.

Acute exposures to neurotoxic agents may have a delayed effect, which further confounds the ability to determine the cause of mental deterioration. At a given threshold of exposure, a certain percentage of brain cells may be destroyed. Less affected cells may be injured and weakened. These cells are then likely to die prematurely, as typical aging patterns and the cumulative assault of other neurotoxic agents continue. Therefore, the cumulative effect of acute or low-level exposures to neurotoxic agents may not be noticed for many years.

The problematical temporal relationship of exposure to neurotoxic agents and onset of symptoms are mentioned by Arrezo and Schaumburg (1989). They pointed out that neurotoxicity symptoms may intensify for months after exposure has stopped (coasting). In another scenario, symptoms may only appear after years of low-level exposure. Even if a person is aware of exposure to toxic chemicals, the onset of symptoms may be insidious and may not be detected by the person affected or by their health professional.

Awareness of the relationship between neurotoxic chemical exposure and such neural diseases as senile dementia (Alzheimer's disease) is hampered by the delayed or cumulative effects of neurotoxicants. We are currently aware that some diseases, such as cancer, caused by asbestos exposure, may take 20 years to develop. Without careful study, the causal connection of asbestos and cancer could have been overlooked. Similarly with neurotoxicity, repeated assaults to neural tissue by many different types of neurotoxic chemicals over many years may weaken the nervous system, thus leading to greater risk of degenerative brain diseases. For example, the risk of Alzheimer's disease or pre-senile dementia may be increased in individuals with significant neurotoxicity. These diseases are diagnosed years after the occurrence of marked deterioration in mental function, and could be related to neurotoxic chemical or drug exposure occurring many years before.[4] Arezzo and Schaumburg (1989) also suggest that neurotoxic damage early in life can increase central nervous system dysfunction in conditions, such as Parkinson's disease, that occur late in life.

In an investigation of lead as a contributing factor to Alzheimer's disease, Niklowitz and Mandybur (1975) examined the brain of a person who had lead-induced CNS dysfunction for 40 years. Brain neuro-fibrillary tangles characteristic of Alzheimer's presenile dementia were found by them.

The Value of "Risk-assessment" for Evaluating the Risk of Neurotoxicity. Risk assessment describes the process by which researchers and policy decision makers determine the risk of disease from exposure to a chemical. In many or most cases when this term is used, the risk that is being quantified is the risk of cancer, and does not include the risk of other diseases and conditions such as neurotoxicity. In a recent textbook on risk assessment, neurotoxicity is not even mentioned in the table of contents or the index (Hallenbeck and Cunningham 1987).

This limitation of risk assessment is not well known. Although cancer is a dreaded disease, other diseases do exist, and they are also unpleasant. This deficiency of risk assessment, as currently practiced, will not soon be remedied, because it is rarely if ever discussed in the general scientific-toxicologic literature (although the September 1989 Seventh International Neurotoxicity Conference addressed this issue; Cranmer, 1989).

The pervasive lack of knowledge regarding neurotoxicity was illustrated by the United States General Accounting Office in their review of the adequacy of risk assessment by the FDA, OSHA, and EPA (GAO, 1987). For example, GAO reviewed FDA's risk analysis for regulating methylene chloride; OSHA's risk analysis for regulating organic arsenic; and EPA's risk analysis for regulating volatile organic compounds. In GAO's *oversight* review they neglected to even mention neurotoxicity risk assessment, although these three substances are notably neurotoxic. This review illustrates a blind spot of government agencies in their effort to protect the American public from toxicity of commercial products. Multiple government agencies did not even consider neurotoxicity when determining the risk of exposure to notably neurotoxic substances.

---

4. The environmental hypothesis for brain diseases is briefly reviewed by Lewin (1987). Spencer et al. (1987) have linked an environmental (food) chemical exposure, occurring many years earlier with no apparent effects, with neural disease occurring at a later date, specifically amyotrophic lateral sclerosis—Parkinsonism—dementia. Spencer thought that other environmental chemicals may also act as triggers for neuronal death (Lewin, 1987). Calne and Spencer speculated that Alzheimer's disease may be due to environmental damage to the central nervous system and that damage may remain subclinical for several decades but makes those affected especially prone to the consequences of age-related neuronal attrition (Lewin, 1987).

Threshold of Effect of Neurotoxic Substances. At present there is little evidence for a threshold effect for many neurotoxic substances. Substances that are inhaled can pass directly into the bloodstream and then to the brain, without passing through the liver detoxification system. The brain itself has few detoxification mechanisms. The brain cells then must react with the potentially toxic substance. With neurotoxic substances, this reaction can damage brain cells. As described above, if a cell does no die, it can become weakened, function less efficiently, and become more susceptible to future damage. Therefore, it is likely that many neurotoxic substances can cause neurotoxicity at very low exposure levels, although the damage may be unnoticeable.

Relationship of Neurotoxicity to Other Diseases

The most serious disease which is commonly attributed to chemical toxicity is cancer. However, toxic chemicals can damage every organ in the body, especially the human nervous system, without causing cancer. Damage to any organ can have ramifications for the central nervous system because of the lowering of the body's ability to maintain optimal function.

Many substances that are neurotoxic are also suspected or known to cause cancer. There substances include benzene, other solvents, pesticides, herbicides, PCBs, dioxines, and formaldehyde. Cancer often takes many years to develop. (Asbestos may have a carcinogenic latency of 20 years.) In contrast, neurotoxicity can often be detected within a much shorter period of time. Acute effects may be noticed immediately, if the dose is high enough, while the chronic effects of low-level exposure can be measured with the appropriate neuropsychological tests. These tests will be described in later chapters. By preventing or limiting neurotoxicity, we may also reduce the risk of cancer.

In addition to causing cancer, many neurotoxic substances can alter the immune system, leading to immune system dysregulation. A number of neurotoxic substances (pesticides, solvents, etc.) have been associated with chemical hypersensitivity. In turn, alterations of the nervous system can affect the immunologic system. The immunologic system, by both identifying and neutralizing toxic substances, and scavaging mutant cells, is intimately involved in the defense against cancer. Psychoneuroimmunology is the term used for the study of the interrelationship of these three functional organic systems. Damage to all three systems can be caused by neurotoxic chemicals.

The immune and nervous systems have a number of similarities. Both receive information from outside and inside the body, and code the information by amplifying specific molecules (the immune system) or encoding in a specific pattern of neuronal firings. Both systems adapt to their environment, and communicate extensively within themselves (Cunningham, 1981).

The nervous and immune systems interact in a complex way. Some of the methods of interaction include the production of corticosteroids and other hormones, which affects immunologic function, and which in turn can be affected by stress or other psychological factors. The hypothalamus is related to immediate and delayed hypersensitivity, while stimulated lymphocytes are believed to have hormone receptors (Cunningham, 1981).

Damage to the nervous system therefore is likely to have ramifications in the immunologic system. A controversial topic is the condition of chemical hypersensitivity. People with this condition apparently have an allergic-type reaction to levels of toxic substances below those which affect normal people. It is thought that the condition arises from toxic chemical derangement of the immune system. Perhaps neurotoxicity plays a causative role in this condition.

In addition to a direct neurophysiologic effect of chemical agents on the immunologic system, a secondary effect can occur because of psychological factors, such as depression and stress over lost mental function, that can result from neurotoxicity.

The neurotoxicity monitoring program that will be described in later chapters provides some protection and reduce the risk of diseases affecting organs other than the nervous system.

Effects of Neurotoxicants on Aging

Percentage of Older People.   The elderly population is growing much more rapidly than the population as a whole. Census projections for the year 2050 indicate that the proportion of the population over 65 will be 22%, compared with 12% today (Siegel and Taeuber, 1986). As discussed elsewhere in this chapter, the percentage of U.S. citizens over the age of 65 with symptoms of dementia is more than 10%. The percentage may be increasing. If the cause of this condition remains constant, the total number of people with dementia will surely grow.

Silent Neurotoxicity May Manifest as Dementia in Later Years.   Exposure to neurotoxic chemicals can cause "silent" brain damage. With silent brain damage, the brain may continue to function adequately, even though brain cells are injured or dying because of neurotoxicity. The brain functions in a way that allows parts of the brain that are uninjured to compensate for an injured part, thereby letting an injury remain unnoticed. However, with continued exposure to toxic chemicals, the reserve capacity of the brain becomes exhausted, resulting in dementia.

Aging allows previously masked neurotoxic disorders to emerge (NAS, 1987). An age-related decline in neural function might allow previously silent neurotoxic disorders to reach clinical expression (Calne et al., 1986).

Nervous system dysfunction occurs after the structural and functional redundancy of the nervous system has been exhausted. For example, Parkinson's disease occurs after considerable loss of the substantia nigra. The destruction of brain cells must reach a certain threshold before the disease state remains constant (NAS, 1987).

The interaction of toxic chemical effects and aging have been proposed as the cause of Alzheimer's type dementia. Subclinical damage of specific regions of the brain, the effects of which become unmasked over the years, can be caused by neurotoxic substances. The specific regions of the brain which are most affected, are those regions most susceptible to toxic substances and age-related neuronal attrition. The unmasking process arises because of many factors that contribute to aging, including the cumulative effects of exposure to neurotoxic substances over the years (Calne et al., 1986).

COSTS OF NEUROTOXICITY

Accidents.   Accidents are the third leading cause of death in the United States (Almanac, 1988). Cardiovascular disease and cancer are the first and second leading causes of death. Because neurotoxicity reduces brain functional ability, it increases the risk of accidents. As mental acuity decreases, the risk of accidents increases. Visual perception, manual dexterity, and short-term memory are all important elements in the causal chain of accidents. As sensory perception becomes impaired, tools may drop, instructions may be forgotten, and attention may be easily distracted.

Accidents are a drain on company expenses and morale. Hospital and medical expenses, worker and disability expenses from accidents amount to many millions of dollars per year. Expenses for lost training and expertise must be counted in the economic impact of accidental death and injury.

Dementia.   Neurotoxicity reduces brain function and can result in the death or weakening of brain cells. The nervous system is then more susceptible to additional toxic insults and disease processes, leading to an increased risk of dementia, such as Alzheimer's disease (Singer, 1988). The symptoms of Alzheimer's disease are indistinguishable from and may actually be identical to those of severe dementia.

Prevalence of Dementia.   Studies of over 3,600 elderly people have found that 10.3% of the sample over age 65 have memory impairment or other mental problems for which the most likely cause is Alzheimer's type dementia (Leary, 1989). For people over 85, 47.2% were diagnosed with the disease. The estimated number of Americans with this disease was 4 million (Evans, 1989).[5]

Researchers have been concerned that dementia among people living outside of nursing homes may be more prevalent than has previously been suspected. Pfeffer (1987) studied 800 people over the age of 65 who were living outside of nursing homes. Subjects were given cognitive and neurological tests that are more sensitive than the usual clinical tests for senile dementia. Dementia was found in 16% of those examined. For subjects over the age of 80, living outside of nursing homes, Pfeffer (1987) found 36% to be demented. From 57% to 78% of nursing home residents are thought to have dementing conditions (OTA, 1987).

Costs of Dementia. In 1987, estimates of the annual expected cost for an Alzheimer disease patient, excluding the value of lost productivity, was about $18,000. The total cost of the disease per patient in 1983, was between $50,000 to $500,000, depending upon the patient's age at disease onset (Hay and Ernst, 1987).

The National Institute of Aging estimated that the annual cost in 1986 for nursing home care for patients with severe dementia was $38 billion. Between $400 and $800 million is spent annually on diagnosis of dementia (OTA, 1987).

Costs for informal home care of demented relatives is estimated at $27 billion. The cost includes lost wages of the caretaker, hiring of additional home care staff, home alterations to increase the patient's safety, etc. (OTA, 1987).

The economic costs for this condition are severe. Another consideration, in addition to economic costs, is the personal tragedy of losing what could be the best years of one's life, by the steady erosion of personality and of the unique characteristics of humanity—memory, language, communication. For families caring for the demented at home, life can become an unending hell, until or unless the patient can be placed in a nursing home.

It is likely that the quantity and quality of brain cells, which do not regenerate, can be eroded by continuous exposure to neurotoxic chemicals in our food, water, and air. The eroded brain is then more susceptible to other conditions or factors that may cause dementia. Based upon my personal research over the past 10 years, examining hundreds of people with neurotoxicity, and

---

5. In 1987, an estimated 1.5 million Americans suffered from severe dementia. An additional 1 to 5 million were estimated to have mild or moderate dementia. The number of people with severe dementia was expected to increase by 60% by the year 2000. About 6% of Americans over 65 were estimated to have severe dementia, with an additional 6-18% showing mild-moderate dementia. (For comparison purposes, in the United States, only 5% of those over 65 have suffered some type of stroke; Kistler, 1989). Prevalence of severe dementia for those over age 85 was estimated at 25% (OTA, 1987).

studying the available research literature, I am convinced that environmental and occupational neurotoxic chemicals can increase susceptibility to or cause dementia. Other researcher's have also voiced opinions about the toxic chemical causes of dementia.

The relationship between dementia and neurotoxicity was raised by Robert Butler (1987), former head of the National Institute of Aging, who stated that a key issue when considering neurotoxicity and aging is the environmental effect of neurotoxic chemicals on the CNS. The CNS is a key pacemaker of aging. Neurotoxic effects are not all-or-nothing effects; as with any toxic impact on the central nervous system, symptoms or effects are produced on a continuum.

These ideas were amplified by Williams et al. (1987), who were concerned that a large proportion of the neurodegenerative diseases in the general population may result from neurotoxic chemicals. They thought that repeated subclinical exposure to neurotoxic substances may augment the already identified age-associated decline in neural integrity, and increase the probability that neurological and psychiatric disorders will surface in old age.

Chemically-induced neurological disorders are often virtually indistinguishable from other causes of disease, suggesting the possibility that environmental chemicals mimic the action of metabolically-generated chemical substances circulating in the blood. The decline of neurologic integrity associated with the aging process might be linked with the cumulative effects of endogenous or exogenous poisons. "Logical pursuit of this line of thought leads to the conclusion that the study of nutrition and toxicology will impact substantially on the knowledge of the biology of neurological aging" and the cause of neurological and psychiatric disorders (Williams et al. 1987).

Generalized Poor Health. The brain and nervous system coordinate the functions of all body organs. When the nervous system deteriorates, such as can occur with neurotoxicity, the health of all the body's organs becomes compromised. Nervous system efficiency is reduced under conditions of neurotoxicity. Because the brain monitors and directs the function and regeneration of the entire body, chronic neurotoxicity can generally increase the risk of other diseases.

General Health Care Costs. The U.S. expenditure for health care amounts to 12% of the Gross National Product (Kramon, 1988). In 1989, an estimated $620 billion will be spent on health care costs. By 1991, Americans will spend $2 billion per day (Califano, 1989). With an estimated population of 280 million, per capita spending will be $2,600 per year. The government picks up the lion's share of health costs, through direct payment for services and indirect costs of research, grants, and other programs.

Early recognition of toxicity is important to taxpayers and to the government.

The burdens of sickness are shared in modern society. Health care costs are a major drain of the GNP in the developed countries. Economic considerations urge us to examine the potential causes of illness and take appropriate preventive measures.

A Public Health Issue of Neurotoxicity

Bellinger et al. (1987) studied the effects of prenatal low-level lead exposure on children's intelligence. The entire range of lead exposure was within the "safety limit" set by the U.S. Center for Disease Control. However, children with more prenatal lead exposure scored 8% lower on a test of mental development than did children with lower prenatal lead exposure. Dr. Bernard Weiss, a founder of the field of behavior toxicology, pointed out the ramifications of this finding. If these findings applied to the general population, the number of persons with superior intelligence would fall from 2.3 million per 100 million to less than 1 million (Moses, 1989). In Dr. Weiss's words, this would be "a societal disaster."

The preceding lead study was conducted on one chemical. Consider the multitude of chemicals to which mothers, infants, and children are exposed, and the magnitude of the public health concerns for neurotoxicity becomes more apparent.

REGULATION OF NEUROTOXICITY

Tilson (1989) reviewed the United States regulatory mandates concerning neurotoxicity. Although the National Institute of Occupational Safety and Health (NIOSH) recognizes that neurotoxicity is a very important cause of occupational disease (CDC, 1983), specific tests of neurotoxicity are not required to evaluate neurotoxicity among workers. This unfortunate oversight does not protect workers from getting sick, nor can management rely upon this oversight to insulate them, and their employers, from lawsuits and other legal actions for neurotoxically-induced injury and disease. This topic will be covered in a later chapter.

The U.S. Environmental Protection Agency has been slow to recognize neurotoxicity as an important problem, and it does not regulate neurotoxins adequately. For example, the U.S. General Accounting Office (GAO, 1986a; 1986b) found that EPA has failed to adequately protect the public from pesticide hazards. Neurotoxicity from gasoline fuels also poses hazards to our citizens: although clean air has been an issue for a number of years, there is little mention of the neurotoxicity of gasoline fuels (Singer, 1987a). In a document entitled *Health Effects Assessment Summary Tables* (EPA, 1989), the EPA attempted to catalogue the toxicity, other than carcinogenicity, of commercial products that it regulates. The EPA failed to recognize neurotoxicity for many neurotoxic substances, including heptachlor, carbon tetrachloride, and other solvents and pesticides.

The U.S. Food and Drug Administration (FDA) does not adequately protect the public from pesticides in food. The tolerances of pesticide residue that are permitted, and the widespread presence of pesticide residue on food was discussed in an earlier section.

Another problem facing the FDA is a lack of adequate staff to enforce the current residue standards. The FDA has 226 district office staff members involved in import inspection tasks. For these tasks, the staff spent, on the average, 38% of their time in paperwork, 13% in travel to inspection sites, and 22% in physical inspection (GAO, 1989a).

FDA inspectors must be on the lookout for chemicals which are banned in the United States, but which are not banned in other countries and which may be on imported produce. Pesticides that have lost their EPA registration because of toxicity continue to be manufactured in the United States and are sent abroad for other countries to use (GAO, 1989b). Unfortunately for U.S. citizens, these pesticides come back to the United States in the form of food, including produce and fruit. The FDA, whose 226 staff members spend 22% of their time inspecting produce at all the points of entry to the United States, may not be looking for unregistered pesticide contaminated produce. This situation does not promote confidence in the safety of our imported produce. Consequently, many U.S. citizens are searching for, and finding produce and other commodities grown without pesticides.

Additional protection gaps can also be found in the U.S. Department of Agriculture and the EPA. The U.S. government bought $15 million worth of apples to reduce a huge surplus that arose when customers stopped buying apples because of concerns about the chemical Alar (also known as diminozide), which is used to make apples ripen uniformly. However, the apples were to be distributed to schools, prisons, food aid programs (poor children, etc.) and others. Although the U.S. EPA plans to ban Alar, which has been linked to cancer in children, the EPA said that there is no danger from apples sprayed with the chemical (AP, 1989). There appear to be a number of contradictions in EPA policy.

The EPA first received evidence that Alar posed a threat of cancer in the mid-1970s but did not announce it's intention to remove the chemical from the market until 1989 (Shabecoff, 1989). At that time, public fear that the chemical could cause cancer caused apple sales to plummet. In draft legislation, EPA stated "the Alar case illustrates that allowing continued use of pesticide products for years after significant health risks are identified results in loss of public confidence in government's ability to protect [the public's] health."

The document also stated that the Alar incident was not an isolated case, and that as the agency examined more evidence about pesticides that have been on the market for many years, it would inevitably find some that presented high risks to health. The EPA is now proposing new rules that would permit the agency to remove dangerous chemicals from our food supply.

Recent Trends at EPA. The policies of the EPA directly reflect the wishes of the presidential administration. Under Ronald Reagan's administration, EPA's role in environmental protection was diminished. However, federal policy in this area seems to be changing.

EPA has recently joined the researchers around the world who for many years have been concerned about indoor air pollution. EPA has found that indoor air pollution is one of the most serious U.S. health problems, and has called for government research and education programs to determine safe exposure levels of a host of chemicals found in homes, offices, and hospitals. Chemicals to be studied included formaldehyde, pesticides, and chlorinated solvents. In a three volume report sent to key members of U.S. Congress, EPA said that indoor pollution costs billions of dollars per year in lost wages, lowered productivity, and medical expenses. Current federal efforts to learn about and act on indoor pollution were termed "almost nonexistent" (Sternberg, 1989).

On another front, EPA appears to be more eager to police agricultural pesticides. On December 4, 1989, EPA proposed a 90% reduction in the use of EBDCs (ethylene bisdithiocarbamate), a widely used class of fungicides, because they are thought to cause cancer. EBDCs have been used since 1935. Eighteen million pounds are now used annually in the United States and more is used abroad (Gold, 1989). Unfortunately, EPA did not appear to offer growers any ideas for alternative farming practices. The two primary chemical replacements for EBDC are captan and chlorothalonil, both of which are reportedly carcinogenic. Will EPA also ban these in the future? And on what grounds will EPA decide?

The EPA's efforts, at present, in investigating agricultural chemicals are primarily focused on cancer. If EPA broaden's it's perspective to other areas, such as neurotoxicity, will chemicals be banned at an increasing rate?

EPA almost seems to be at war with the Department of Agriculture, which promotes the use of chemicals in farming. Conflict arises because changes in the understanding of toxicology and the public's perception of risk causes EPA to respond, and this response conflicts with federal farm policy. At some point, EPA, the Department of Agriculture, and other federal agencies should form a rational policy regarding the whole issue of pesticide toxicology and farming practices and needs.

Ironically, the National Academy of Sciences has found that farmers who apply little or no chemicals to crops can be as productive as those who use pesticides and synthetic fertilizers, and the Academy recommends changing federal subsidy programs that encourage overuse of agricultural chemicals

(Schneider, 1989). Many farmers are already growing food without toxic chemicals, using techniques known as permaculture, sustainable agriculture, organic farming, and natural farming. These practices promote environmental health and land productivity.

REFERENCES

Aguayo, Albert J. 1987. Regeneration of axons from the injured central nervous system of adult mammals. In *Encyclopedia of the Brain*, Vol. 1, George Adelman, ed. Boston: Birkhauser.

Almanac. 1988. *The World Almanac and Book of Facts*. New York: Pharos Books.

Anger, W. K. 1986. Workplace exposures. In *Neurobehavioral Toxicology*, Zoltan Annau, ed. Baltimore: Johns Hopkins University Press.

Anger, W. K. 1984. Neurobehavioral testing of chemicals: Impact on recommended standards. *Neurobeh. Toxicol. Teratol.* 66:147–53.

Anger, W. K. and Johnson, B. 1985. Chemicals affecting behavior. In *Neurotoxicity of Industrial and Commercial Chemicals*. Vol. 1, J. O'Donoghue, ed. Boca Raton, Florida: CRC Press.

Associated Press. 1989. Government will buy apples left over from scare on Alar. *New York Times*. January 7, 1989.

Arezzo, Joseph C. and Schaumburg, Herbert H. 1989. Screening for neurotoxic disease in humans. *J. Am. Coll. Toxicol.* 8(1):147–55.

Bellinger, David; Leviton, Alan; Waternaux, Christine; Needleman, Herbert and Rabinowitz, Michael. 1987. Longitudinal analysis of prenatal and postnatal lead exposure and early cognitive development. *N. Engl. J. Med.* 316(17):1037-43.

Bondy, Stephen. 1988. The neurotoxicity of organic and inorganic lead. In *Metal Neurotoxicity*. Stephen Bondy and K. Prasad, eds. Boca Raton, Florida: CRC Press.

Broad, William J. 1981. Sir Isaac Newton: Mad as a hatter. *Science* 213:1341–44.

Butler, Robert. 1985. Keynote Address, Workshop on environmental toxicity and the aging process, October 1, 1985. In *Environmental toxicity and the aging process*. Scott R. Baker and Marvin Rogul, eds. New York: Alan R. Liss.

Califano, Joseph A., Jr. 1989. *New York Times*, p. A25, April 12, 1989.

Calne, D. B.; McGeer, E.; Eisen, A. and Spencer, P. 1986. Alzheimer's disease, Parkinson's disease, and motoneurone disease: Abiotropic interaction between ageing and environment? *Lancet* 2:1067–70.

CDC. 1986. Prevention of leading work related diseases and injuries. *Morbidity and Mortality Weekly Report*, 35(Feb. 28, 1986).

CDC. 1983. Leading work related injuries and diseases—United States. *Morbidity and Mortality Weekly Report*, 32(8):24–26.

Cooper, J. R., Bloom, F. E., and Roth, R. M. 1986. *The Biochemical Basis of Neuropharmacology*, 5th Ed., Oxford University Press: New York.

Cranmer, Joan. 1989. Seventh International Neurotoxicology Conference, *Fund. and Applied Toxicol.*, 13:181.

Cunningham, Alastair J. 1981. Mind, body and immune response. In *Psychoneuroimmunology*. Robert Ader, ed. New York: Academic Press.

Ecobichon, D. and Joy, R. 1982. *Pesticides and Neurological Diseases*, CRC Press: Boca Raton, Florida.

EPA. 1989. *Health Effects Assessment Summary Tables*. Third Quarter, FY 1989. OERR 9200.6-303-(89-3), July 1989.

EPA 1976. Core activities of the office of Toxic Substances (Draft Program Plan), EPA Publication 560/4-76-005, Washington. Cited in Landrigan, P. J.; Kreiss, K.; Xintaras, C.; Feldman, R. G. and Clark, W. H. 1980. Clinical epidemiology of occupational neurotoxic disease. *Neurobeh. Toxicol*. 2:43-48.

Evans, Denis A. 1989. *J. of the Am. Med. Assoc.*, November 10, 1989.

Friedman, Robert. 1981. *Sensitive Populations and Environmental Standards*. Washington, D.C.: The Conservation Foundation.

Fulkerson, William; Reister, David B.; Perry, Alfred M. et. al. 1989. Global warming: An energy technology R&D challenge. *Science*, 246:868-9.

GAO. 1989a. *Imported Foods: Opportunities to Improve FDA's Inspection Program*. United States General Accounting Office, GAO/HRD-89-88, April 28.

GAO. 1989b. *Pesticides: Export of Unregistered Pesticides is Not Adequately Monitored by EPA*. United States General Accounting Office, GAO/HRD-89-128, April 25.

GAO. 1987. *Health Risk Analysis: Technical Adequacy in Three Selected Cases*. The United States General Accounting Office, GAO/PEMD-87-14, September 1987.

GAO. 1986a. *Pesticides: EPA's Formidable Task to Assess and Regulate Their Risks*. United States General Accounting Office, GAO/RCED-86-125.

GAO. 1986b. *Nonagricultural Pesticides: Risks and Regulations*. United States General Accounting Office, GAO/RCED-86-89.

Gold, Allan R. 1989. Tight limits proposed for popular farm chemicals. *New York Times*, A20, December 5, 1989.

Hallenbak, W. H. and Cunningham, K. M. 1987. *Quantitative Risk Assessment for Environmental and Occupational Health*. Chelsea, Michigan: Lewis Publishers.

Hartman, David. 1988. *Neuropsychological Toxicology*. Pergamon Press: New York.

Hay, Joel W. and Ernst, Richard L. 1987. The economic costs of Alzheimer's disease. *Am. J. Pub. Heal*. 77(9):1169-75.

Hershko, H. et al. 1984. Lead poisoning in a West Bank Arab village. *Arch. Int. Med*. 144:1969-73.

Iyaniwara T. 1990. Mammalian toxicity and combined exposure to pesticides. *Vet. and Hum. Toxicol*. 21(1):58-62.

Johnson, Barry L. Ed. 1987. *Prevention of Neurotoxic Illness in Working Populations*. Chichester, England: John Wiley & Sons.

Katzman, R. 1981. Blood-Brain-CSF barriers. In *Basic Neurochemistry*, 3rd ed. G. Siegel et al. eds. Boston: Little Brown and Company.

Kistler, Philip. 1989. How can we prevent strokes? *Harvard Medical School Health Letter*, 14:10. August 1989.

Koshland, Daniel E., Jr. 1989. Solar power and priorities. *Science*, 245(4920):805. August 25, 1989.

Kramon, Glenn, 1988. Business and health: Important issues to watch in 1989. *New York Times*, D2, December 27, 1989.

Landrigan, Philip J. 1988. Lead: Assessing it's health hazards. *Health and Environment Digest*, 2(6):1-2.

Landrigan, Philip J., Kreiss, Kathleen, Xintaras, Charles, Feldman, Robert G. and Heath, Clark W. Jr. 1980. Clinical epidemiology of occupational neurotoxic disease. *Neurobehav. Toxicol.* 2(1):43–8.

Leary, Warren E. 1989. New study increases the estimate of the frequency of Alzheimer's disease. *New York Times*, p.A1. November 10, 1989.

Lewin, Roger. 1987. Environmental hypothesis for brain diseases strengthened by new data. *Science*, 237:483–484. July 31, 1987.

Moses, Susan. 1989. Food coloring may alter kid's behavior. *APA Monitor*, p. 9, October, 1989.

NAS. 1987. *Aging in Today's Environment*. National Research Council, Washington, D.C.: National Academy Press.

Niklowitz, W. J. and Mandybur, T. I. 1975. Neurofibrillary changes following lead encephalopathy. *J. Neuropathol. Exp. Neurol.* 34:445–55.

National Research Council. 1986. *Drinking Water and Health*. National Academy Press, Washington, DC.

NIOSH. 1977. Springfield, Virginia: National Technical Information Service; Publication No. PB-82-229881.

NRDC. 1984. *Pesticides in Food: What the Public Needs to Know*. San Francisco: National Resources Defense Council. March 15, 1984.

Oldendorf, William. 1987. The blood-brain barrier. In *Encyclopedia of Neuroscience*, Vol. 1, George Adelman, ed. Boston: Birkhauser.

OTA. 1987. Losing a million minds: Confronting the tragedy of Alzheimer's disease and other dementias. US Congress, Office of Technology Assessment, OTA-BA-323, Washington, D.C.: U.S. Government Printing Office, April, 1987.

Pfeffer, R. I., Afifi, A. A., and Chance, J. M. 1987. Prevalence of Alzheimer's disease in a retirement community. *Am. J. Epidemiol.* 125(3)420–436.

Proctor, Nick H.; Hughes, James P., and Fischman, Michael L. 1988. Chemical Hazards of the Workplace, 2nd ed. Philadelphia: Lippincott.

Richter, Elihu. 1988. Personal communication.

Rose, F. Clifford. 1987. Headache. In *Encyclopedia of the Brain*, Vol. 1, George Adelman, ed. Boston: Birkhauser.

Schneider, Keith. 1989. Science academy recommends resumption of natural farming. *New York Times*. p. A1. September 8, 1989.

Schneider, M. J. 1979. *Persistent Poisons*. New York: New York Academy of Sciences.

Shabecoff, Philip. 1989. E. P. A. proposing quicker action against suspect farm chemicals. *New York Times*. p. 1A. July 20, 1989.

Siegel, J. S. and Taeuber, C. M. 1986. Demographic perspectives on the long-lived society. *Daedalus*, 115(1):77–117.

Singer, R. (in press, 1990) Nervous system monitoring for early signs of chemical toxicity. *Biological Monitoring of Exposure to Metals*. New York: John Wiley & Sons.

Singer, R. 1990. Neurotoxicity can produce "MS-like" symptoms. *Journal of Clinical and Experimental Neuropsychology*. 12(1):68.

Singer, R. (1988). Early recognition of toxicity by assessing nervous system function. *Biomedical and Environmental Sciences*, 1:365–362.

Singer, R. 1987a. *The Toxicity of Gasoline Additives*. Unpublished report.

Singer, R. 1987b. How to prove nervous system dysfunction. *A Guide to Toxic Torts*. New York: Matthew Bender.

Singer, R., Valciukas, J., and Lilis, R. 1983. Lead exposure and nerve conduction velocity: The differential time course of sensory and motor nerve effects. *Neurotoxicology*, 4(2):193–202.

Smith, Marjorie. 1986. Lead in history. In *Lead Toxicity*. Richard Landsdown and William Yule, Eds. Baltimore: Johns Hopkins University Press.

Spencer, P. S., Nunn, P. B., Hugon, J. et al. 1987. Guam amyotrophic lateral sclerosis—Parkinsonism—dementia linked to a plant excitant neurotoxin. *Science*. 237:517–522.

Sternberg, Ken. 1989. EPA pegs indoor air as health threat. *Chemical Week*, p. 9. August 16, 1989.

Tilson, Hugh A. 1989. Introduction screening for neurotoxicity: Principles and practices. *J. Am. Coll. Toxicol.* 8(1):13–17.

Valciukas, J.; Lilis, R.; Singer, R.; Glickman, L. and Nicholson, W. J. 1985. Neurobehavioral changes among shipyard painters exposed to solvents. *Archives of Environmental Health*, 40(1):47–52.

Wedeen, R. P. 1984. Poison in the Pot: The Legacy of Lead. Carbondale, IL: Southern Illinois University Press.

Weiss, Bernard. 1986. Emerging challenges to behavioral toxicology. In *Neurobehavioral Toxicology*, Zoltan Annau, ed. Baltimore: Johns Hopkins University Press.

WHO. 1986. Principles and Methods for the Assessment of Neurotoxicity Associated with Exposure to Chemicals. Environmental Health Criteria 60. Geneva.

Williams, Jerry R.; Spencer, Peter S.; Stahl, Stephen M. et al. 1987. Interactions of aging and environmental agents: The toxicological perspective. In *Environmental Toxicity and the Aging Process*, pp. 81–135. Scott R. Baker and Marvin Rogul, eds. New York: Alan R. Liss.

2

EVALUATION OF NEUROTOXICITY

INTRODUCTION

For a number of reasons the nervous system offers opportunities to monitor the possibly harmful effects of chemicals on living humans.

1. The nervous system is relatively accessible to measurement through the sense organs. It is the interface between the internal organs and the outside world. Hence, the observer can communicate with the body through the sense organs. This allows a quick and intelligent evaluation of organ system function.

2. A wide range of organ response within each function is possible because of the complexity of the nervous system function. This permits extensive quantification of organ function, which is an important aspect of the measurement of human functions.

3. The functions that the nervous system can perform are practically limitless, and therefore many different functions can be measured to give a broad picture of the organism's response to toxicity.

4. Functional deficits are directly relevant to human decision-making. In contrast, the measurement of levels of chemicals in blood, fat or other tissue may be of unknown significance. Imaging of brain anatomy is also of limited use in many or most cases of neurotoxicity, because currently available techniques may not be sensitive to effects at the cellular level, and wide variations of response between individuals can occur even with similar appearing physical injuries.

5. Sophisticated and time-tested procedures are available to measure both central and peripheral neural processes.

6. The nervous system is particularly sensitive to dysfunction caused by chemical toxicity. The brain is the most highly evolved organ of which man is aware, and has been termed "The Crown of Creation." Efficient nervous system function depends upon a complex net of biochemical and bioelectrical interactions about which scientists are only beginning to learn. Reactive chemicals that are foreign to the chemical environment in which the brain has evolved appear to interfere with brain function when they come in contact with the organ.

7. Because of the sensitivity and complexity of the brain, toxicity affecting

practically any organ can influence brain function. As organ system function decreases because of toxicity, the brain's ability to support general body function diminishes. For example, as pulmonary function decreases, less oxygen may be available to the brain. As cardiac function decreases less fresh blood may be available for brain tissues. Minor toxicity of more than one organ system can have a multiplicative effect on nervous system function.

8. Brain nerve cells do not regenerate, therefore damage from neurotoxic chemicals can be both permanent and cumulative. To prevent permanent and cumulative damage to the nervous system, it is important to catch the earliest signs of chemical toxicity affecting this organ.

BIOLOGICAL MONITORING

Biological monitoring is the term used to describe the assessment of chemical exposure by measuring biological activity, in contrast to the environmental measurement of chemicals in air, water, soil, etc.* The lowest level of biological monitoring involves sampling of the chemicals or their metabolites in blood, urine, expired air, fat, or hair. The next level of biological monitoring involves measurements of a biological effect, such as changes in liver function, but the significance of these measurements may be unclear. Alterations in biological indicators may reflect benign physiological variations or an adverse health effect. An effect is considered adverse if it impairs functional ability or capacity in a significant way.

The main advantage of the biological monitoring of adverse health effects over environmental monitoring is that biological monitoring can evaluate functional changes in an individual. People vary from each other in chemical uptake, metabolism, biotransformation and excretion of toxic substances (Lauwerys, 1984).

Many safety programs rely upon monitoring of air, water or dust to determine the safe levels of a substance. This approach has been criticized because it does not take into account the variable dosages that individuals may receive, depending upon factors such as duration of exposure, route of exposure, and biological activity. Biological monitoring (BM) arose in an attempt to access the "internal dose" of an environmental pollutant. In contrast to environmental monitoring, BM attempts to account for both external total exposure and individual variability (Zielhuis, 1984).

In review of BM, Zielhuis (1984) pointed out that outcome measures of BM programs should distinguish between effects caused by short term exposure and effects due to long term exposure. He indicated that BM programs designed to

---

*Baselt (1988) describes analytical methods for biological monitoring. Information about these techniques appears in a journal called *Biological Monitoring: An International Journal*, published by Telford Press, Caldwell, New Jersey.

evaluate short-term exposure effects may not be suitable for evaluating long-term effects. Long-term, low-level exposures may have different effects, particularly on organ systems such as the human brain, that do not regenerate cells. Zeilhuis was also concerned with the validity of BM data, which is often "too poor" and therefore can be misleading. BM has been studied for metals where the reliability of the data was too low for use. Unacceptable error rates have occurred both within and between laboratories measuring equivalent samples of blood spiked with lead.

Blood Tests.   Blood tests can determine the presence of substances in the blood. The tests are usually specific for a particular chemical. If the person being tested is exposed to more than one chemical, or if the number of possibly neurotoxic chemicals to which an individual is exposed is unknown, this type of testing becomes impractical.

Blood tests for foreign substances in the blood must be carried out within a limited time. Red blood cells, which comprise more than 99% of blood volume, are replaced every 120 days (Guyton, 1981). Therefore, the information gathered by measuring foreign substances in blood is limited by time.

Fat Biopsy and Other Body Tissue Sampling Techniques.   It is possible to extract fat and body tissues for examination of traces of toxic substances. This approach can cover a wider span of time than can blood samples. However, the techniques are more invasive, and may be resisted by people who need to be monitored on frequently. A problem raised above for blood tests also arises when considering tissue sampling—which substances should be measured? Even if the examiner knows that a person has been exposed to PCB, which type of PCB should be measured? Which type is more toxic? What about impurities of other substances that may be extremely toxic, such as dioxin? These are difficult questions.

Another problem with this approach arises because the significance of the presence of low levels of toxic substances in body tissue is not clear. Does the substance have an impact on health when present in low concentrations? Where is the best location to search for body burdens of toxic chemicals? Many toxic substances are soluble in fat; the brain and nerves use fat as insulation. However, low levels of toxic substances in fat from the buttocks may not reflect the levels of toxic substances in brain fat. Low levels of toxic materials in fat may mean that other molecules of the substance have had the opportunity to travel through the body and create injury, while lesser amounts have been stored in fat for more gradual release. Conversely, high levels in buttock fat may reflect a shifting of the substance from neutral fat to safer fat locations, for more gradual release into the blood. These possibilities reduce the applicability of such means for monitoring neurotoxicity.

Hair Chemical Analysis.   According to Laker (1982), chemical analysis of hair holds promise for the monitoring of exposures for the following reasons:

1. Hair provides a better assessment of normal trace element concentrations because short-term variations are averaged out. By taking a piece of hair equivalent to a few weeks growth and measuring the bulk concentration, an average concentration over that period may be found.

2. Hair offers a good way of discerning long-term variations in trace element concentrations. This may be done by measuring the variations along the length hair that has been growing for several months, or by taking samples periodically.

3. Unlike blood, hair is an inert and chemically homogeneous substance. The structure of hair is permanent and once a trace element atom is incorporated into it, the element is fixed there.

4. The concentrations of most trace elements are relatively high in hair compared to the rest of the body, especially blood.

5. Hair provides a record of past as well as present trace element levels.

6. Specimens can be collected more quickly and easily than specimens of blood, urine, and any other tissue. Specimens do not deteriorate and may be kept indefinitely without the need for special storage considerations.

However, at the present time, there are a number of problems concerning the validity of hair chemical analysis.

1. In addition to systemic intoxication, chemicals in the hair may be caused by chemicals falling on the hair from external sources. It is difficult to distinguish the source of the contamination from hair analysis, so high levels may not reflect systemic intoxication.

2. The normal concentrations of elements in hair has not been established. This factor is less relevant when repeated measurements are used to monitor chemical exposure.

3. There may be a lack of standardized approaches to preparing the hair for analysis and conducting the analysis. Again, this factor is less relevant when repeated measurements, using the same procedures, are used to monitor chemical exposure.

4. Researchers are not sure how or to what extent substances are incorporated into hair; some toxic substances causing systemic intoxication (i.e., solvents) may not be deposited into hair. Hair analysis for metal toxicity seems to be a more reliable application of the technique (Chatt and Katz, 1988).

Evaluation of early myelotoxicity, hepatotoxicity and nephrotoxicity, monitoring of mutagenicity in urine, and evaluation of chromosomal aberrations are beyond the scope of this book. For a discussion of these topics see Aitio et al. (1984). However, clinical dysfunction caused by such conditions will probably have an effect on the central nervous system, causing the symptoms of neurotoxicity.

For further discussion of the early detection of occupational diseases, see WHO (1986a). This book presents a short discussion and evaluation of nervous system function and covers measurement of other organ systems. For a general discussion of chemical hazards in the workplace see Proctor et al. (1988). For a general discussion of the clinical toxicology of commercial products see Gosselin et al. (1984).

Imaging Techniques. Imaging techniques describe the methodology used to visually portray the anatomy and neurophysiology of tissue that is surrounded by skin and—in the case of the brain—hair, skin, and bone. The techniques used are x-ray, including computer-assisted tomography (CAT) scan, positive emission tomography, (PET) scan and other radioactive scans, and magnetic resonance imaging (MRI) (Bigler et al. 1989).

Ruff et al. (1989) compared the sensitivity of CAT, MRI, and PET scans with neuropsychological testing. Because CAT and MRI scans provide only a static view of neural structure, their usefulness is limited. In six head injury cases, CAT and/or MRI scans yielded little or no evidence of neuropathology as detected by neuropsychological testing. PET scans, however, corroborated the impaired function.

Imaging techniques are often of little value in neurotoxicity evaluations (Arezzo and Schaumburg, 1989). In my experience and those of others, imaging can occasionally pick up abnormalities, but in general, symptoms and behavioral deficits can occur without imaging-located defects. Imaging techniques are not suitable for routine screening because they are expensive and may pose health risks.

Biochemical Methods for Neurotoxicological Analysis. Although in the future, it may be possible to develop methodologies for measurements taken from blood or urine, or exhaled air, which would reliably precede the onset of neurotoxicity, until that time, testing for nervous system function is needed.

Ho and Haskins (1989) provide a description of the biochemical methods used in neurotoxicological research. The methods were not necessarily proposed for biological monitoring.

Behavioral Toxicology. Behavioral Toxicology describes the science of evaluating the effects of chemicals on behavior. The term applies to both animal and human studies. Johnson and Anger (1983) reviewed the history of the field of human behavioral toxicology. The first textbook in the field was edited by Weiss and Laties (1975). Its application to health monitoring is discussed below. Recent reviews of animal behavioral toxicology can be found in Norton (1989) and WHO (1986b).

MONITORING NERVOUS SYSTEM FUNCTION

Monitoring nervous system function provides an excellent approach to determining the early effects of toxic substances on human health. This type of measurement is more immediately valid, meaningful, and significant than many other types of monitoring. Monitoring of functions provides an early warning for the onset of disease.

Nervous system function can be monitored with tests that evaluate nervous system function that require input from the subject (psychometric tests) or neurophysiological measures that rely more upon bio-electric functioning. Psychometric tests are constructed to measure functions including memory, concentration, reaction time, manual dexterity, and other psychological or neuropsychological functions. Although both approaches have merit at the present time, it appears that the most sensitive, meaningful, and cost-effective method of evaluation of neurotoxicity developed to date is the psychometric test.

Hanninen (1984) reviewed behavioral methods for the assessment of early impairments in central nervous system function. Behavioral methods include the evaluation of symptoms and the use of psychometric tests to elicit behavior that can be measured and compared with normal or control values. Hanninen reviewed studies of lead, inorganic mercury, and organic solvent using behavioral methods and found that behavioral methods are useful for the prevention of disease in conjunction with more direct methods of biological monitoring. Behavioral methods can be used as a substitute for biological monitoring when no adequate methods for biological monitoring are available, for example, in multiple chemical exposures.

Hanninen (1984) pointed out some aspects of behavioral methods that require attention for the accurate assessment of neurotoxicity.

1. There may be large variations of psychological functions because of normal fluctuations in such functions. This limitation can be reduced by taking baseline measurements.

2. False positive findings can be found even when baseline performances are known. Therefore, when a worker is identified by screening approaches, a more thorough examination is recommended. Another approach would be to examine the effects at a group level.

These matters will be discussed in the chapter describing monitoring programs.

The limitations pointed out by Hanninen (1984) illustrate the need for professional psychological expertise when planning behavioral methods for health surveillance. However, if properly planned, the testing may be carried out by trained occupational nurses or similar personnel.

Symptom Screening. On logical grounds, symptom screening is probably the single most effective approach to determining the earliest signs of neurotoxicity. Significant alterations in function will probably be reported if the subject is questioned. Questionnaires take very little time to administer and score.

One limitation of symptom screening is the lack of sensitivity to very subtle levels of neurotoxicity. Another limitation, similar to screening approaches for any disease, is the possible lack of specificity of the screen. For a more comprehensive approach to detecting neurotoxicity, see Chapter 3.

A questionnaire approach to the monitoring of early disturbances of central nervous system function was explored by Hogstedt et al. (1984). These investigators found testing for symptoms to be valuable for determining the adverse effects of some occupational exposure situations. Other researchers, from time to time, have published papers on the use of symptom questionnaires in neurotoxicity research.

Limitations of some questionnaires may include the lack of quantification of the frequency or severity of the impairment. Usually, the questions are answered in a yes or no fashion, which may not accurately reflect this situation. A person may have symptoms rarely or frequently; this makes a difference in the total health impact of the disease, if the disease is present.

Another limitation of questionnaires can be the limited range of symptoms that are included. Neurotoxicity can affect many types of nervous systems function, so a wide variety of symptoms should be covered.

A third limitation of some symptoms questionnaires is the lack of description of which types of symptoms are most prominent. This limitation can be overcome by the determination of factor scores for various nervous system functions.

The Neurotoxicity Screening Survey (NSS) (Singer, 1990: Singer and Scott, 1987a) was developed to provide total quantification of the frequency, type, and severity of neurotoxicity symptoms. Frequency is determined by a rating scale, ranging from ''never'' to ''most of the time.'' Type is determined by combining symptoms with in functional groups, such as memory, peripheral numbness, and sensory-motor function. Severity is determined by the global score. Figure 2-1 shows sample neurotoxicity symptoms probes.

DESCRIPTION OF THE NEUROTOXICITY SCREENING SURVEY

The NSS is a 121 item symptom questionnaire constructed with a 5 point Likert Scale. Symptoms were drawn from the pool of neuropsychological symptoms in the literature (Hogstedt et al. 1984; Lezak, 1983; Melendez, 1978; PAR,

The following is a list of items that describes how you may have been feeling lately. Please rate each item as accurately as possible, and do not skip any items.

1	2	3	4	5
Never	Rarely	Sometimes	Often	Most of the time

1. Memory problems		1 2 3 4 5
2. Concentration problems		1 2 3 4 5
3. Short attention span		1 2 3 4 5
4. Can't think as quickly as before		1 2 3 4 5
5. Difficulty thinking clearly		1 2 3 4 5
6. Easily distracted		1 2 3 4 5
7. Trouble starting on tasks		1 2 3 4 5
8. Trouble planning ahead		1 2 3 4 5
9. Trouble with "common sense"		1 2 3 4 5
10. Trouble following a conversation		1 2 3 4 5
11. Trouble remembering the right word when talking		1 2 3 4 5
12. Trouble understanding others		1 2 3 4 5
13. Get lost		1 2 3 4 5
14. Forget time and day		1 2 3 4 5
15. Forget where you are		1 2 3 4 5
16. Forget what someone tells you		1 2 3 4 5
17. Periods where you "lose" time		1 2 3 4 5
18. Momentary blank or inattentive spells		1 2 3 4 5
19. Forget meetings		1 2 3 4 5
20. Forget things that happened after a few hours		1 2 3 4 5
21. Forget things that happened after a few minutes		1 2 3 4 5
22. Forget where you are going		1 2 3 4 5
23. Forget where you placed objects		1 2 3 4 5
24. Trouble understanding what you read		1 2 3 4 5
25. Forget what you read		1 2 3 4 5
26. Forget mental math		1 2 3 4 5
27. Trouble telling right from left		1 2 3 4 5
28. Trouble getting dressed		1 2 3 4 5
29. Trouble driving		1 2 3 4 5
30. Forget your name for a few hours		1 2 3 4 5
31. Headaches		1 2 3 4 5
32. Sleep problems		1 2 3 4 5
33. Overly drowsy		1 2 3 4 5

Figure 2-1. Sample Neurotoxicity Screening Survey symptom probes.

1983; Schinka, 1984; Singer, 1987; Singer and Scott, 1987a; Valciukas et al, 1985;1980). This symptom pool was reduced by selecting those symptoms that have been reported to be common among workers and patients suffering from neurotoxicity.

Results are scored in 11 categories: Autonomic Nervous System, Balance, Chemical Sensitivity, Distortion, Emotionality, Hearing, Memory-Concentration, Peripheral Numbness, Sensory-Motor, Smell-Taste, and Vision. An overall neurotoxicity indicator is also provided. Results are compared with responses of people with diagnosed neurotoxicity. Figure 2-2 shows a sample report sheet.

The NSS is self-administered, and takes about 20 to 30 minutes to complete. A sixth grade reading level is required.

The distortion factor consists of symptoms that are physiologically improbable. The citing of these symptoms raises the question of symptom distortion or malingering.

Validation

The NSS was administered to 36 subjects with diagnosed neurotoxicity and 33 subjects without unusual exposure to neurotoxic chemicals or diagnosed neurologic disorders. The controls subjects included students from a New York City university; workers from Texas; various older individuals from Philadelphia and Miami; and staff at a psychotherapy practice in Washington, D.C. From the available completed protocols, the control subjects were selected if they reported: no known toxic exposure, little or no recreational drug use, and no diagnosed neurological disorder.

Mean Analysis. The exposed and control subjects were closely matched by age and education; no significant difference was found upon t-test analysis of these variables (Table 2-1).

Mean values on the ten symptom factors, and the overall neurotoxicity indicator, were compared for the exposed and control groups (Table 1-1). Significant differences were found on every factor.

Discriminant Analysis. Using the algorithm of classifying subjects as neurotoxicity indicator score fell within 1.5 standard deviations of the mean for the study group, 89% of the controls and 86% of the study group were correctly classified.

Multiple Correlation Analysis. The multiple correlation of the factors with group status was found to be 0.90, $p < .0000001$. The adjusted R square was 0.74. These results show that symptom quantification of the NSS is highly correlated with group membership.

Reliability. The general Kuder-Richardson formula for determining reliability of the overall neurotoxicity indicator wa calculated, using Cronbach's formula for generalizing dichotomous and non-dichotomous scores (Guilford and Fruch-

Patient's name:_____

Date of test:_____

Factor	Normal	Elevated
	(check one)	

Memory and Concentration_____

Autonomic Nervous System _____

Vision_____

Hearing_____

Balance_____

Smell-Taste_____

Peripheral Numbness_____

Sensory-Motor_____

Chemical Sensitivity_____

Emotionality_____

Distortion_____

Overall Neurotoxicity Indicator_____

If the Overall Neurotoxicity Indicator is elevated, the patient reported symptoms similar to those reported by patients with diagnosed neurotoxicity.

If any factor scores are elevated, the patient reported more frequent and bothersome symptoms in these categories than that occurs in most people without illness or unusual exposure to neurotoxic chemicals.

Figure 2-2. Neurotoxicity Screening Survey: Clinical Report.

ter, 1978). The reliability coefficient for the overall neurotoxicity indicator was 0.86

Versions B.   Version B is identical to Version A, with addition of response rows for "Before Exposure"; "Right after Exposure"; and "Past 6 Months."

Table 2-1. Mean analysis of neurotoxic patients compared with non-exposed controls[1]

Variable	N	Mean	Std. Dev.	t	Prob. t
Age					
Patients	36	43.0	10.2	−.58	0.56
Controls	33	44.9	15.7		
Education					
Patients	36	12.7	2.1	−1.28	0.21
Controls	33	13.5	2.8		
Memory Concentration					
Patients	32	3.02	0.69	10.86	<.0000001
Controls	30	1.49	0.40		
Autonomic Nervous System					
Patients	25	2.72	0.64	8.33	<.0000001
Controls	31	1.50	0.39		
Vision					
Patients	35	1.94	0.78	5.46	.0000003
Controls	33	1.17	0.30		
Hearing					
Patients	34	2.76	1.26	6.37	.0000001
Controls	33	1.29	0.46		
Balance					
Patients	36	2.64	1.31	6.89	<.0000001
Controls	33	1.09	0.29		
Smell Taste					
Patients	36	2.34	1.13	6.22	.0000003
Controls	33	1.14	0.26		
Peripheral Numbness					
Patients	35	2.85	1.04	9.49	<.0000001
Controls	33	1.13	0.23		
Sensory-Motor					
Patients	34	5.53	1.90	9.74	<.0000001
Controls	32	2.28	0.40		
Chemical Sensitivity					
Patients	30	2.78	1.25	6.73	.0000001
Controls	33	1.17	0.43		
Emotionality					
Patients	36	3.03	0.85	6.98	.0000001
Controls	31	1.84	0.56		
Distortion					
Patients	33	1.71	0.72	5.39	.0000006
Controls	33	1.03	0.11		
Neurotoxicity Indicator					
Patients	21	27.9	7.27	8.81	<.0000001
Controls	26	13.1	2.82		

1. Factor scores are divided by the mean number of variables in each factor so that the factors can be compared with each other.

This version is especially useful for evaluation of forensic cases and for cases where symptom change from before exposure to after exposure in important.

Limitations of the NSS.   Elevated scores on the NSS may not always mean that neurotoxicity is present. This is a limitation of many laboratory and psychological tests. Like perhaps all medical or psychological tests, results of the NSS must be interpreted by a skilled clinician who can determine if other factors may have contributed to elevated scores.

The distortion factor is not as reliable as the other factors. People with neurotoxicity have distortion of nervous system responses. Because of the number of unusual sensations they may experience, they are more likely to respond positively to the symptom probes that describe unusual or unlikely sensations. Some of the distortion questions have been reworded so that true positive responses are less probable.

A number of additional distortion questions which are less based upon sensory experience, but more based upon psychological experience, have been added to the questionnaire. However, neurotoxicity can also distort psychological experience, so the examiner cannot rely solely upon these or any responses to determine that the person is deliberately distorting his responses.

At present, the added distortion questions do not increase the distortion factor score, but the added responses can be used for clinical purposes to evaluate distortion. These probes have been drawn from Rogers (1988), who described methods to evaluate malingering and deception. Based primarily on theoretical grounds and clinical experience, symptoms such as those described in these questions are unlikely in illness that is being truly reported. If responses to these questions are affirmative, the examiner should be concerned that the respondent may be malingering or distorting.

Although the individual probes may not offer certain proof of distortion, deception and malingering, when the distortion probes are answered affirmatively, it would be prudent to look carefully at the subject's responses. Does a pattern of responding positively to distortion questions emerge? Does the person offer a credible reason for checking the probes? Was the person confused when responding to the questionnaire? At this point, clinical judgement comes into play.

PSYCHOMETRIC TESTING

There are many psychometric tests in print. Lezak (1983) admirably reviewed the psychometric tests used in neuropsychology. An introduction to neuropsychological assessment is provided by Hartlage et al. (1987). In practice, the tests that are selected depend upon the requirements of the situation. For neurotoxicity screening, tests need to be selected which provide the most information in the shortest period of time. Such tests also should be reliable and valid. Test selection depends upon the judgement and experience of the examiner. Some neuropsychologists prefer to use the same battery of tests for all patients.

Batteries of Psychometric Tests

Halstead-Reitan. Among neuropsychologists who use a pre-selected battery, the Halstead-Reitan Battery is the most widely used neuropsychological set of tests (Goldstein, 1984). It contains about 12 subtests. Although sections of the test may be applicable to neurotoxicity screening, a test of this length would be too costly to administer on a routine basis.

WHO Neurobehavioral Core Test Battery. The World Health Organization (WHO) and the US National Institute of Safety and Health (NIOSH) proposed a core battery of tests to be applied to neurobehavioral research around the world (WHO, 1986c; Johnson, 1989). This battery included the following:

Test	Functional Domain Tested
Profile of Mood States	Affect
Simple Reaction Time	Attention/Response Speed
Digit Span	Auditory Memory
Santa Ana Dexterity Test	Manual Dexterity
Digit Symbol	Perceptual-Motor Speed
Benton Visual Retention Test	Visual Perception/Memory
Pursuit Aiming	Motor Steadiness

The test is now being administered around the world to determine its suitability and norms. The battery takes about 45 to 60 minutes to administer.

Helsinki Neurobehavioral Test Battery (Hanninen and Lindstrom, 1988). Helena Hanninen pioneered the use of neurobehavioral tests for evaluating occupational and environmental toxicity (Hanninen, 1985). Along with other Nordic scientists an clinicians, Hanninen has published on a number of investigations of various neurotoxic substances. Many test from this battery are used for individual neuropsychological examinations for neurotoxicity.

Pittsburgh Occupational Exposures Battery (POET) (Ryan et al. 1987). The POET is a 90-minute battery of tests drawn from tests which were sensitive to neurotoxic effects. It includes several subtests from a WAIS-R and Wechsler Memory Scale, as well as a number of learning, memory, visuospatial, and visuomotor tests. Norms were gathered on 182 blue-collar workers recruited from a heavy industrial plant that manufactured auto and truck chassis. Subjects were screened for previous exposure to heavy metals, mixtures of organic solvents, and toxic inhalants. Equations were constructed to predict scores on the basis of age and education. The battery has been successfully applied to groups with neurotoxic chemical exposure (Morrow et al. 1987).

Neurobehavioral Evaluation System (NES) (Baker et al. 1985). The NES is a battery of tests that are designed to be administered with a microcomputer. The selected tests are similar to the tests found in the WHO battery described above. Computerized tests have the advantages of lower administration costs and the ability to perform some tests that are otherwise difficult to administer. The NES is the most widely used computer battery in neurotoxicity research.

Before computerized human neurotoxicity testing becomes widely accepted, a number of issues will have to be settled. (1) As with all psychometric testing, the subject must be closely watched (while the tests are administered) to determine the validity of the testing procedure. (2) A possibly uncontrolled variable of computerized testing is the amount of experience that a population might have had with computers and keyboards. Many working class men have no experience with such equipment, and may not perform optimally and in a valid way on a computerized battery of tests. Other subjects may have an extensive experience with keyboards or computer games, and may therefore have inflated scores. (3) Subjects may find computers to be boring to interact with, and may become restless and hurry to terminate the proceedings.

These factors can be closely monitored when human testing is performed an a human administrator is present. Further research may help clarify the possibly confounding effects of these factors.

Individual Neuropsychological Testing for Neurotoxicity

There are many psychometric tests that could be used to evaluate nervous system dysfunction. Neuropsychologists often use comprehensive batteries (See Goldstein, 1984 and Lezak, 1983 for critiques of comprehensive batteries). However, when evaluating neurotoxicity within a limited period of time, selecting of tests for sensitivity to neurotoxicity provides a more efficient approach to assessment than simply using a prepackaged, comprehensive battery. Test selection is based upon the cumulative experience of psychologists around the world who study problems of neurotoxicity.

A standard component of my neurotoxicity examination and that of a large number of neuropsychologists in the United States is the Wechsler Adult Intelligence Scale, Revised (WAIS-R) (Wechsler, 1981). This test is composed of subtests that evaluate mental functions including vocabulary, information, psychomotor reaction time, visuospatial perception, and logical thinking. The test protocol and norms are well standardized, and the statistical properties of the scores are well documented. The WAIS-R provides a rich source or neuropsychologic information in a relatively short period of time. In addition to quantitative data, qualitative information is provided by observing the process by which the subject completes assigned tasks.

Additional tests were selected primarily for their sensitivity to the type of deficits found with neurotoxicity.

1. The revised Benton Visual Retention Test (Benton, 1974) shows deficits in short-term visual memory and is easy to administer and score.

2. Recent memory is evaluated with paragraphs from the Wechsler Memory Scale (Wechsler, 1972; Wallace, 1984).

3. The Embedded Figures Test (Valciukas and Singer, 1982) screens for deficits in figure-ground visual perception.

4. The Army Trailmaking Test (described in Lezak, 1983) measures concentration and mental flexibility. Additional norms for this test can be found in Bornstein (1985).

5. The Grooved Pegboard Test measures manual dexterity. This test is described in Lezak (1983) with additional norms in Bornstein (1985).

6. The Dot Counting Test and the Memorization of 15 Items (Lezak, 1983) may be used to test malingering.

7. The Paced Auditory Serial Addition Test (Lezak, 1983) and the Stroop Color-Word Test (Golden, 1978) measure mental flexibility and concentration.

8. The Controlled Oral Word Association Test (Lezak, 1983) measures the ability to find words.

9. The Expanded Paired Associate Learning Test measures recent and delayed memory (Trahan et al. 1989).

10. The Profile of Mood Scale (McNair et al. 1981) and the Beck Depression Scale (Beck and Steer, 1987) evaluate emotional function.

11. The Neurotoxicity Screening Survey, described above in this chapter, evaluates symptoms.

Deficit Measurement Paradigm. It is exceedingly rare for the average subject to have had the identical tests administered prior to exposure to the toxic chemical. Typically the neuropsychologist must determine the presence of any mental deficits by an examination after the exposure. If deficits are found, how can it be ascertained that the deficits did not exist prior to exposure? In most cases, the earlier level of functioning must be estimated. The *deficit measurement paradigm* was developed for such situations (Lezak, 1983).

Pre-exposure function is estimated from different types of data, including school records, standardized tests, employment testing and records, military testing and records, and other historical data. Honors, awards or other evidence of achievement can supply helpful information. Within this framework, the present level of function is compared with an estimate of premorbid ability to determine the presence of deficits.

Because diffuse brain damage of recent or adult origin does not affect all mental functions similarly, current performance on specific functions can also be used to estimate premorbid ability. Pre-exposure function can be estimated by examining performance on functions known to be resistent to neurotoxic effects, such as vocabulary and long-term memory functions. Well-learned skills, such as vocabulary or information, are less affected by toxic chemical insults, while learning of new materials, required for recent memory and complex problem-solving, is more vulnerable. Performance on tasks more susceptible to toxicity are compared with performance on tasks which are less susceptible to ascertain if the characteristic pattern of neurotoxicity is present.

Oral or written descriptions from people who were familiar with the subject prior to exposure can provide background that is helpful in determining changes in mental and emotional function, and in personality. Information from co-workers, employers, acquaintances, and relatives of the patient may also be useful.

Examples of the individual neurotoxicity testing procedure can be found in Singer (1987); Singer and Scott (1987b); and in Chapter 5.

NEUROPHYSIOLOGICAL TESTS

Neurophysiological tests offer the advantage of somewhat greater objectivity than is offered by tests that require a person to respond. However, up to the present time they lack the sensitivity and manifest meaningfulness of behavioral methods.

Electroencephalogram (EEG).   EEG measures the electrical activity of the brain, by using electrodes placed on the scalp and amplifying the electrical signal for display, usually as lines on paper. EEG is generally not used in neurotoxicologic research as it lacks sensitivity, although it is widely used in clinical settings. EEG abnormalities can be seen as waveform asymmetries when comparing the two brain hemispheres; increased activity of the slow brain waves; or unusually sharp waves or spikes. Abnormalities may be diffuse or localized in one hemisphere or a part of the brain (Johnson, 1987). Some uses of EEG in neurotoxicological research were presented by LeQuesne (1987).

Brain Evoked Potentials (EP).   Measurement of brain evoked potentials is similar to measurement of EEG, but EP uses a sensory signal to begin the measurement period and to provide a standardization stimulus. For example, when measuring touch EP (somatosensory evoked potential), an electrical shock may be presented to the hand. The onset of the shock begins measurement of brain electrical activity. In this fashion, responses of the brain to standardized stimulation can be assessed. The EP can be analyzed for latency of response (how long it takes for the sensory input to travel the nervous system to a specified location of the brain); quantity of response (how strong a signal results); and quality of response (similarity of the EP to normal responses).

EP is used to assess subjects who cannot otherwise communicate (animals, infants, the retarded, or the comatose), and subjects with possible disease processes, such as multiple sclerosis (MS). MS has been found to alter EP, even when more common test, such as visual acuity, remain normal (Squires and Ollo, 1986).

An introduction to evoked potential recording procedures is presented by Squires and Ollo (1986). The basic elements of the system are stimulus delivery equipment, differential amplifiers, and a computer for averaging EPs. The waveform can be analyzed in terms of components, identified by peaks and valleys. The onset of these components indicate the time it takes for the brain to receive information. Latency and amplitude of response is measured at the expected location of normal components of the EP. Latency of response is more reliable than amplitude of response, as latency, compared with amplitude, varies less between subjects.

As the EP stimulus is processed by the brain, certain standard components of the resulting waveform have been identified and agreed upon by many researchers of EP. Exogenous components are components that directly reflect external stimulation, while endogenous components are determined by the subject's interaction with the stimulus.

Auditory EP can be divided into: (1) responses of the brainstem; (2) mid-latency, which seem to come from the auditory cortex; and (3) long-latency, which appear to arise from multiple brain sources, such as the auditory cortex and the thalamus. Auditory EP is used to localize tumors in the auditory system, and is also used to evaluate diseases such as MS (about half of MS patients have abnormalities of auditory EP) (Squires and Ollo, 1986).

Somatosensory EP measures the brains response to electrical, tactile, and kinesthetic stimulation. Limb temperature and body size affect responses. This measure is sensitive to diseases such as MS which affect the conduction of impulses from the peripheral nerves (Squires and Ollo, 1986).

Visual EP is a frequently studied phenomena. Various types of stimulation can be used, including flashes of light, a reversing checkerboard, and a sinusoidal grating (Otto, 1986).

Otto (1986) reviewed the use of sensory EP in occupational medicine. He found that these measures are ideally suited for monitoring the effects of neurotoxic chemicals. Morrow et al. (1988) have applied EP to evaluate exposure to various neurotoxins. They used exogenous and endogenous components of EP, and have found the procedure to be efficacious.

Peripheral Nerve Testing.   The most widely used neurophysiological measure of neurotoxicity is peripheral nerve conduction velocity (NCV) testing. This procedure has been applied to hundreds of studies of neurotoxicity around the world for several decades. NCV testing has been found to provide fairly reliable and valid data.

NCV measures the time it takes for nerve impulses to travel in the arms and legs. The technique is non-invasive, quick, and objective. Electrical activity in the limb is monitored while the nerve is stimulated with an electrical pulse, and the resulting nerve response wave form is both displayed and stored for measurement. Slowing of response or reduced amplitude indicate that the nerve function is impaired. This technique has been used for many years, by many different researchers, to study both normal nerve function and nerves affected by many toxic substances.

For an example of the use of this technique within the context of biological monitoring for metal exposure, see Singer (in press). This chapter discusses the application of NCV to evaluating subclinical metal toxicity. Specific aspects of the techniques will be described in the next chapter. Also see Kimura, 1989 and Ma and Liveson, 1983 for a description of NCV assessment, and Singer et al. 1987; 1983; 1982, for additional examples of the use of NCV assessment in toxicology.

NCV determines the integrity of peripheral nerves by evaluating the latency and amplitude of nerve response (as described above for EP). Often the evaluated nerves include the median motor and median sensory nerves, in the arm and hand, and the sural nerve in the calf. Figure 2-3 shows the NCV setup for evaluating the sural nerve. S indicates the location of the stimulus; Gd represents the grounding electrode; Ra represents the recording electrode; and Rr represents the reference electrode.

Figure 2-4 shows another view of sural NCV measurement. Stimulation is via a small electrical pulse. As the pulse is delivered, the electrical activity under the sensing electrodes is displayed as a waveform (Figure 2-5). The latency of response is reflected by a lack of electrical activity under the sensing electrodes; this is displayed as a relatively flat line (between the two vertical arrows, Figure 2-5). As the nerve receives the signal, it depolarizes, and its electrical activity is temporarily charged negatively (Figure 2-5, peak amplitude).

The choice of the nerves to be monitored for neurotoxicity is very important, according to the following selection factors: (1) The sensory nerves seem to be more sensitive than the motor nerves to neurotoxicity, as reflected by slower

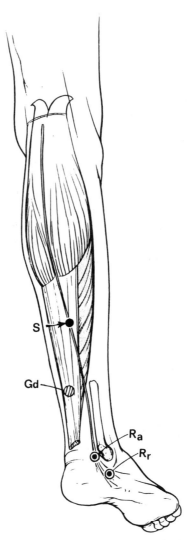

Figure 2-3. NCV setup for evaluating the sural nerve. S indicates the location of the stimulus; Gd represents the grounding electrode; R_a represents the recording electrode; and R_r represents the reference electrode. From Ma, D. M. and Liveson, J. A. 1983. *Nerve Conduction Handbook*. Philadelphia: F. A. Davis. Reproduced with permission.

conduction velocity and reduced amplitude of response; (2) The more distal the nerve segment, the more likely that the nerve will show deterioration, apparently in response to most neurotoxic agents. This condition probably arises because of the physiologic difficulty of maintaining nerve nutrition and metabolism in the long segments of nerve from the nerve cell body at the spine to the

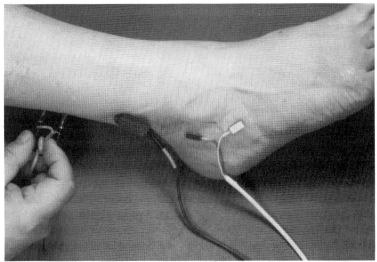

Figure 2-4. Another view of sural NCV measurement, with electrodes (nerve stimulator, ground and sensing electrodes).

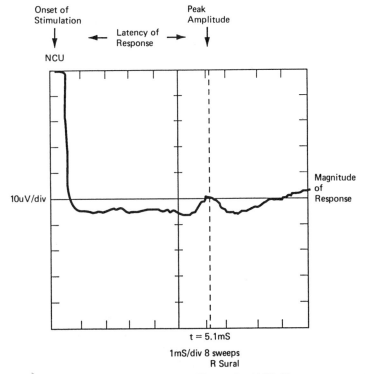

Figure 2-5. Sample NCV wave form. From Singer, R. 1987. Nervous system: Early detection for chemical hazards. *Professional Safety*. March 1987. Reproduced with permission.

nerve endings in the toes or fingers; and (3) the nerves to be selected should produce a clear, easy to obtain and reliable reading.

Sensory nerves of the leg are the logical choice for monitoring peripheral neurotoxicity. The sural nerve has been used by many researchers and clinicians to evaluate neurotoxicity, and is recommended at this time for monitoring programs.

REFERENCES

Aitio, Antero, Riihimhki, Vesa and Vainio, Harri. 1984. *Biological Monitoring and Surveillance of Workers Exposed to Chemicals*. Washington D.C.: Hemisphere Publishing Corp.

Arezzo, Joseph C. and Schaumburg, Herbert H. 1989. Screening for neurotoxic disease in humans. *J. Am. Coll. Toxicol.* 8:(1)147–55.

Baker, E. L.; Letz, R. E.; Fidler, A. T.; Shalat, S.; Plantamura, D. and Lyndon, M. 1985. A computer-based neurobehavioral evaluation system for occupational and environmental epidemiology: Methodology and validation studies. *Neurobeh, Toxicol. Teratol.* 7:369–78.

Baselt, Randall C. 1988. *Biological Monitoring Methods for Industrial Chemicals*, 2nd Ed. Littleton, MA: PSG Publishing Co.

Beck, Aaron T. and Steer, Robert A. 1987. *Beck Depression Inventory*. San Antonio, TX: Psychological Corporation, Harcourt Brace Jovanovich.

Benton, A. L. 1974. *The Revised Visual Retention Test*. 4th Ed. New York: Psychological Corporation.

Bigler, E. D., Yeo, R. A. and Turkheimer, E. eds. 1989. *Neuropsychological Function and Brain Imaging*. New York: Plenum Press.

Bornstein, R. A. 1985. Normative data on selected neuropsychological measures from a nonclinical sample. *J. of Clin. Psych.* 41:5.

Chatt, Amares and Katz, Sidney A. 1988. *Hair Analysis: Applications in the Biomedical and Environmental Sciences*. New York: VCH Publishers.

Golden, Charles J. 1978. *Stroop Color and Word Test*. Chicago: Stoelting Company.

Goldstein, Gerald. 1984. Comprehensive neuropsychological assessment batteries. In *Handbook of Psychological Assessment*, Gerald Goldstein and Michel Herson, eds. Elsmford, NY: Pergamon Press.

Gosselin, Robert E., Smith, Roger P., Hogge, Harold T. 1984. *Clinical Toxicology of Commercial Products*, 5th Ed. Baltimore: Williams and Wilkins.

Guilford, J. P. and Fruchter B. 1978. *Fundamental Statistics in Psychology and Education*. 6th Ed. McGraw-Hill: New York.

Guyton, Arthur. 1981. *Textbook of Medical Physiology*. Philadelphia: Saunders.

Hanninen, Helena. 1984. Behavioral methods in the assessment of early impairments in central nervous function. In *Biological Monitoring and Surveiling of Workers Exposed to Chemicals*. Aitio, Antero; Riihimhki, Vesa and Vainio, Harri, eds., Washington, D.C.: Hemisphere Publishing Corp.

Hanninen, Helena 1985. Twenty-five years of behavioral toxicology within occupational medicine: A personal account. *Amer. J. of Ind. Med.* 7:19-30.

Hanninen, Helena and Lindstrom, Kari 1988. *Neurobehavioral Test Battery of the Institute of Occupational Health.* Helsinki.

Hartlage, Lawrence C.; Asken, Michael J. and Hornsby, J. Larry 1987. *Essentials of Neuropsychological Assessment.* New York: Springer.

Ho, I. K. and Hoskins, Beth. 1989. Biochemical methods of neurotoxicological analyses of neuroregulators and cyclic nucleotides. In *Principles and Methods of Toxicology,* 2nd Ed. A. W. Hayes, ed. New York: Raven Press.

Hogstedt, Christer; Anderson, Kjell and Hane, Monica. 1984. A questionnaire approach to the monitoring of early disturbances in central nervous functions. In Aitio, Antero; Riihimhki, Vesa and Vainio, Harri. eds. *Biological Monitoring and Surveillance of Workers Exposed to Chemicals,* Washington D.C.: Hemisphere Publishing Corp.

Johnson, Barry L., ed. 1989. *Prevention of Neurotoxic Illness in Working Populations.* Chichester, England: John Wiley & Sons.

Johnson, Barry L. and Anger, W. Kent. 1983. Behavioral toxicology. In *Environmental and Occupational Medicine,* William N. Rom, ed. Boston: Little Brown and Company.

Kimura, Jun. 1989. *Electrodiagnosis in Diseases of Nerve and Muscle: Principles and Practice,* 2nd Ed. Philadelphia: F. A. Davis.

Laker, M. 1982. *Lancet,* July 31, 260–62. Found in Chatt, A. and Katz, S. A. 1988. *Hair Analysis: Applications in the Biomedical and Environmental Sciences.* VCH Publishers: New York.

Lauwerys, R. R. 1984. Objectives of biological monitoring in occupational health practice. In Aitio, Antero; Riihimhki, Vesa and Vainio, Harri. eds. *Biological Monitoring and Surveillance of Workers Exposed to Chemicals,* Washington D.C.: Hemisphere Publishing Corp.

LeQuesne, Pamela M. 1987. Clinically used electrophysiological end-points. In *Electrophysiology in Neurotoxicology.* Herbert E. Lowndes, ed. Boca Raton, FL: CRC Press.

Lezak, M. 1983. *Neuropsychological Assessment,* 2nd Ed. New York: Oxford University Press.

Ma, Dong M. and Liveson, Jay A. 1983. *Nerve Conduction Handbook.* Philadelphia: F. A. Davis.

McNair, Douglas M.; Lorr, Maurice and Droppleman, Leo F. 1981. *Profile of Mood States.* San Diego: Educational and Industrial Testing Service.

Melendez, Fernando. 1978. *Adult Neuropsychological Checklist.* Odessa, FL: PAR.

Morrow, L. A.; Kiss, I.; Hodgson, M. J. and Durrant, J. D. 1988. Neurophysiological changes in adults following exposure to neurotoxins. Paper presented to the World Health Organization, December 1988. Washington, D.C.

Morrow L. A. Ryan, C. M.; Stein, D. and Parkinson, D. K. 1987. Neuropsychological deficits in workers exposed to a mixture of organic solvents. *The Clinical Neuropsychologist* 1:88 (Abstract).

Norton, Stata. 1989. Methods for behavioral toxicology. In *Principles and Methods of Toxicology,* 2nd Ed. A. A. Hayes, New York: Raven Press.

Otto, David A. 1986. The use of sensory evoked potentials in neurotoxicity testing of workers. *Seminars in Occupational Medicine,* 1(3):175–183. New York: Thieme Medical Publishers.

PAR. 1983. *Neuropsychological Symptom Checklist.* Odessa, FL: PAR.

Proctor, Nick H.; Hughes, James P. and Fischman, Michael L. 1988. *Chemical Hazards of the Work Place*, 2nd Ed. Philadelphia: J. P. Lippincott Co.

Rogers, Richard, ed. 1988. *Clinical Assessment of Malingering and Deception*. New York: Guilford Press.

Ruff, R. M.; Buchsbaum, M. S.; Troster, A. I.; Marshall, L. F.; Lottenberg, S.; Somers, L. M. and Tobias, M. D. 1989. Computerized tomography, neuropsychology and positive emission tomography in the evaluation of head injury. *Neuropsychiatry, Neuropsychology, and Behavioral Neurology* 2:2.

Ryan, C. M.; Morrow, L. A.; Bromet, E. J. and Parkinson, D. K. 1987. Assessment of neuropsychological dysfunction in the workplace: Normative data from the Pittsburgh Occupational Exposures Test Battery. *J. Clin. Exper. Neuropsychol.* 8(6):665–79.

Schinka, John. 1984. *Health Problems Checklist*. Odessa, FL: PAR.

Singer, R. (in press) Nervous system monitoring for early signs of chemical toxicity. In *Biological Monitoring of Exposure to Chemicals: Metals*, H. Kenneth Dillion and M. Ho eds. New York: John Wiley & Sons.

Singer R. 1990. *The Neurotoxicity Screening Survey*. Raymond Singer, Ph.D.: West Nyack, New York.

Singer, R. 1988. Methodology of forensic neurotoxicity evaluation: PCB case. *Toxicology*, 49:403–408.

Singer, R. 1987. Nervous system: Early detection for chemical hazards. *Professional Safety*, pp. 37–41.

Singer, R. and Scott, N. E. 1987a. Computerized screening for human neurotoxicity by questionnaire: Preliminary results of the neurotoxicity screening survey. *Journal of the American College of Toxicology*, 6(6) (abstract).

Singer, R. and Scott, N. E. 1987b. Progression of neuropsychological deficits following toluene diisocyanate exposure. *Archives of Clinical Neuropsychology*, 2(2):135–144.

Singer, R.; Valciukas, J. and Rosenman, K. D. 1987. Peripheral neurotoxicity in workers exposed to inorganic mercury compounds. *Archives of Environmental Health*, 42 (4):181–184.

Singer, R,; Valciukas, J. and Lilis, R. 1983. Lead exposure and nerve conduction velocity: The differential time course of sensory and motor nerve effects. *Neurotoxicology* 4(2):193–202.

Singer, R.; Moses, M.; Valciukas, J.; Lilis, R. and Selikoff, I. J. 1982. Nerve conduction velocity studies of workers employed in the manufacture of phenoxy herbicides. *Environmental Research* 29:297–311.

Squires, Nancy and Ollo, Christine. 1986. Human evoked potential techniques: Possible applications to neuropsychology. In *Experimental Techniques in Human Neuropsychology*. H. Julia Hannay ed. New York: Oxford University Press.

Trahan, D. E.; Larrabee, G. L.; Quintana, J. W.; Goethe, K. E. and Willingham, A. C. 1989. Development and clinical validation of an expanded paired associate test and delayed recall. *Clin. Neuropsych*. 3(2):169–83.

Valciukas, J.; Lilas, R.; Singer, R.; Glickman, L. and Nicholson, W. J. 1985. Neurobehavioral changes among shipyard painters exposed to solvents *Archives of Environmental Health*, 40(1):47–52.

Valciukas, J.; Lilas, R.; Singer, R.; Fischbein, A.; Anderson, H. A. and Glickman, L.

1980. Lead exposure and behavioral changes: Comparisons of three occupational groups with different levels of lead absorption. *American Journal of Industrial Medicine*, 1:421–462.

Valciukas, J. and Singer, R. 1982 The embedded figures test in epidemiological studies of environmental neurotoxic agents. *Environmental Research* 28:183–198.

Wallace, John L. 1984. Wechsler memory scale. *Internat. J. of Clinical Neuropsychol.* 4:3.

Wechsler, David. 1981. *Wechsler Adult Intelligence Scale*. Revised. New York: The Psychological Corporation.

Wechsler, David. 1972. *Wechsler Memory Scale*. New York: The Psychological Corporation.

Weiss, B. and Laties, V. 1975 *Behavioral Toxicology*. New York: Plenum Press.

WHO. 1986. *Early Detection of Occupational Diseases*. Geneva: World Health Organization.

WHO. 1986b. *Principles and Methods for the Assessment of Neurotoxicity Associated with Exposure to Chemicals*. Environmental Health Criteria 60. Geneva: World Health Organization.

WHO. 1986c. *Field Evaluation of WHO Neurobehavioral Core Test Battery*. Geneva: World Health Organization.

Zielhuis, R. L. 1984. Theoretical and practical considerations in biological monitoring. In *Biological Monitoring and Surveilling of Workers Exposed to Chemicals*. Aitio, Antero; Riihimhki, Vesa and Vainio, Harri, eds. Washington D.C.: Hemisphere Publishing Corp.

3

MODEL NEUROTOXICITY SCREENING PROGRAM

OVERVIEW OF NEUROTOXICITY PREVENTION PROGRAMS[1]

Product Warnings. Through consultation with a neurotoxicologist, companies can determine which substances or products have the *potential* to cause neurotoxicity. Product labels can then be developed which describe the known, potential hazards in simple language.

Employee Monitoring for Neurotoxicity. The simplest and perhaps most cost-effective approach to assess the early effects of neurotoxicity in workers would be symptom evaluation by questionnaire. A screening device such as the *Neurotoxicity Screening Survey* (described in Chapter 2) could be administered on a regular basis. Workers whose symptoms have increased could be further evaluated by health professionals.

Symptom screening may miss some workers who are affected by neurotoxicity because either the screening tests or the individual may be insensitive to the subtle changes that neurotoxicity can cause. Objective tests using psychometric techniques can detect subtle decreases in mental function. Psychometric testing includes testing of reaction time, concentration, memory, perception, manual dexterity, and other functions. It can be completed in less than 20 minutes, with some additional time required for scoring and interpretation.

Neurophysiological testing offers additional low-cost methods for neurotoxicity screening. The test which is most widely available is the nerve conduction velocity test, which evaluates the speed and the strength of nerve response. The testing of two nerves, such as the sural nerves in the calves, could also be completed in 20 minutes by a technician, with some additional time required for scoring and interpretation.

---

[1] The concept of the neurotoxicity prevention program has developed over the past few years, and has been described in part in Singer, in press; Singer, 1988a, and presented at a number of national and international professional conferences (Singer, 1988b; 1986a; 1986b; 1986c; 1985a; and 1985b).

PURPOSES OF THE NEUROTOXICITY SCREENING PROGRAM

1. *Protection of the worker.* When neurotoxicity from occupational exposures first appears, the effects are more likely to be reversible.

2. *Protection of the company.* Reduced civil and criminal liability, lower rates of accidents, lower disability and medical costs.

APPLICATIONS OF NEUROTOXICITY SCREENING PROGRAMS

1. *Pre-employment screening.* Workers should be screened for nervous system function *before* employment, to determine their baseline level of functioning. If problems arise in the future, companies can look at the baseline data to determine if changes in nervous system function have occurred.

2. *Periodic examinations.* Workers should be screened every 6 to 12 months for neurotoxicity.

3. *Selection of affected workers for education and treatment.* Workers with neurotoxicity can be taught better ways to work in potentially hazardous environments. Those severely affected can be referred for treatment.

4. *Early detection of industrial hygiene problems.* The presence of neurotoxicity means there is an industrial hygiene problem. If a cluster of affected workers is found, a problem of neurotoxicity exposure may be more readily identified and located.

DESIGN OF A MODEL NEUROTOXICITY SCREENING PROGRAM

Design of a model neurotoxicity screening program should consider the following factors:

1. *Flexibility.* Companies can select the elements most appropriate for their purposes. Each component will be independent of the other components.

2. *Economy.* Testing procedures should be inexpensive so they can be widely applied.

3. *Speed.* Each procedure should be completed rapidly to keep costs low and facilitate subject compliance.

4. *Brevity.* The tests should be as short as possible, to both reduce costs and increase subject compliance.

5. *Sensitivity.* The tests should be sensitive to the early effects of neurotoxicity.

6. *Easily scored.* It should be possible to score the tests using simple rules, requiring little technical judgement. This reduces the possibility of error.

7. *Quantifiability.* The results should be fully quantified, without qualifying variables. All effects of all variables should be reflected in the final score.

8. *Validity.* The tests should have the demonstrable capacity of measuring what they are supposed to measure (in this case, diffuse nervous system dysfunction). They should have been used successfully in both research and clinical settings in the past.

9. *Reliability.* The tests should be capable of consistent measurement.

10. *Repeatability.* A potential problem with psychometric testing is the alteration of the subject by the testing procedure itself, due to learning. Retesting should present little distortion of results.

11. *Portability.* If tests can be readily assembled, disassembled and transported, this will ease administration of the tests and lower costs.

12. *Robust.* Testing materials should not be overly sensitive to environmental changes, such as temperature, humidity, electrical fields, mechanical pressure (accidental dropping).

13. *Enjoyability.* The testing procedure should be as pleasant as possible, to increase subject compliance.

14. *Professional acceptability.* Tests that are widely accepted in their field are more likely to withstand the scrutiny of legal examination.

15. *Technology.* Low-technological testing often has the advantages of lower testing costs, lower start-up costs, greater reliability (as less can go wrong), and reduced training demands. Although computerized testing may be appropriate as research continues, a more conservative approach relies upon more traditional testing techniques.

16. *Data analysis.* Sensitivity of the testing procedure can be increased by pooling the data and analysing the data as a group to magnify small changes. This will help address problems while they are still small and manageable.

STATISTICAL ASPECTS OF NEUROTOXICITY SCREENING PROGRAMS

Normative Interpretations of Scores.   If baseline data is not available, the subject's scores will have to be compared with the scores of people of similar age, sex, and education levels. These standard values are available in the literature.

Deficit Measurement Paradigm.   This concept, discussed in Chapter 2 enables the examiner to determine if a significant variation from chance performance has occurred. For example, vocabulary scores, which are resistant to neurotoxicity, can be compared with scores that measure more sensitive functions, such as memory and concentration.

Standard Error of Measurement.   All measurements contain some error. Even the use of a yardstick produces some variation from measurement to measurement over time, depending upon temperature, humidity, the skill of the person using the yardstick, etc.

All psychological test results approximate the ideal "true" score. Each test has a known ability to approximate the "true" score. This ability is called the standard error of measurement (SEM) or the standard error of a score, which reflects the average deviation of scores from the theoretically true scores. The SEM is defined as the standard deviation of the test scores multiplied by the square root of one minus the reliability of the test scores (McNemar, 1969) (Figure 3-1). Reliability is defined as the correlation between two comparable measures of the same thing, i.e., two administrations of the same test (test-retest reliability).

Difference Scores.   To determine that a true difference in scores has occurred, the interpreter must consider the test reliability and error of measurement. For example, a difference of five or more points may or may not be statistically meaningful. The standard error of a difference score equals the square root of the sum of the square of the SEM of each measure (Anastasi, 1989) (Figure 2).

The statistical treatment of psychological test data has been developed for many years. Sources of information include Anastasi (1988), McNemar (1969), and Guilford and Fruchter (1978). Psychological test data is routinely used by scientists, medical and psychology clinicians, and the legislative and legal systems. Shuman (1986) and Blau (1989; 1984) discuss the legal acceptance of psychological data.

MODULES OF NEUROTOXICITY SCREENING PROGRAMS

It is highly recommended that a licensed psychologist supervise the administration and interpretation of psychometric tests. There are many factors which may be important for correct application of the recommended procedures that cannot be covered entirely in this book. Depending upon state law, it may be illegal

$$SEM = S_x \sqrt{1 - r_{xx}},$$

where

SEM = Standard Error of Measurement
S_x = Standard Deviation of the Measurement
r_{xx} = Reliability of the Measurement.

Figure 3-1. Standard error of measurement.

$$SE\,\text{difference} = \sqrt{\left(SEM_1\right)^2 + \left(SEM_2\right)^2}$$

where

$SE\,\text{diff}$ = Standard Error of the Difference between Two Scores
SEM_1 = Standard Error of Measurement of First Administration of Test
SEM_2 = Standard Error of Measurement of Second Administration of Test

Figure 3-2. Standard error of a difference score.

for psychological tests to be administered without the supervision of a licensed psychologist, or it may be unethical for a health professional with a different license to supervise the administration of psychological tests. To help insure appropriate professional cooperation testing procedures should be planned with an occupational health physician, or with a local physician who is a available for consultation.

Symptom Screening. The symptoms of neurotoxicity were covered in Chapter 1. The Neurotoxicity Screening Survey (NSS) can be self-administered, and takes 5 to 10 minutes to complete (see Chapter 2). Scoring and interpretation of each NSS takes about 5 minutes, and can be done by a clerk. The clerk must be adequately supervised by a licensed mental health professional, to ensure competence and professional handling of sensitive mental health data. The questionnaire can be computerized, but this extra step may not be necessary.

The cutoff scores for normals versus neurotoxically-affected individuals can be used to detect abnormalities. A more sensitive approach to determine statistically meaningful changes in symptomatology of retested individuals would be to calculate the difference score and determine if the value is statistically significant. These calculations can easily be done with personal computers using statistical and database packages.

Psychometric Testing. The following tests are useful for neurotoxicity screening. They do not all have to be administered. If funds are very limited, the Digit Symbol Test is recommended.

1. *Digit Symbol Test* (Wechsler, 1981). This test requires the subject to write down a symbol in a row of blocks below a row of numbers (Figure 3-3). This test assesses psychomotor speed, complex reaction time, and short-term memory. It takes a few minutes to administer and score the test. This test appears to be the most sensitive one available for detecting diffuse brain dysfunction, such as occurs with neurotoxicity.

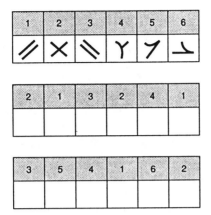

Figure 3-3. Example of the digit-symbol coding task. From Lezak, M.D. 1983. *Neuropsychological Assessment*. New York: Oxford University Press. Reproduced with permission.

In contrast to most psychometric tests, this test can be administered in a group situation, greatly reducing administrative costs. (The Trails Test, described below, can also be administered in a group). When the results are interpreted, if a baseline measure is not available, due consideration should be given to age and educational background of the subjects. The simultaneous administration of a vocabulary test can help the interpretation by providing a measure of education.

The Symbol Digit Modalities Test (Smith, 1973) is similar to the Digit Symbol Test, but has the possible advantage of reversing the task by requiring the subject to write in (or call out) the number that is associated with each digit. This test is suitable for those who cannot write.

2. *Digit Span Test* (Wechsler, 1981). This is a test of the ability to remember spoken numbers, and is designed to measure the span of immediate verbal recall. The test requires about five minutes to administer, and is very easy to score. It includes the challenge of repeating numbers in the reverse direction (digits backwards), which requires the ability to remember the numbers and mentally manipulate the order (mental tracking). Digits backwards appears to be more sensitive than digits forward to subtle brain dysfunction.

When administered to patients, this test may not be sensitive to subtle brain damage. However, its validity may be increased when a baseline measurement is available. Simplicity is a reason for its inclusion in a screening battery.

A variation of the Digit Span Test measures the ability to recall a string of eight or more random numbers. Described as a "rote learning task," in contrast to digit span (an "immediate memory task"), this test has been used to detect memory disorders (Benton et al. 1983). Whether this test is more successful than the measure of digits backwards is uncertain.

Digit span could be administered in a group situation, with the subjects writing their responses in pen, and erasures not permitted. Because artifacts may be introduced, this administrative variation may be more appropriate when baseline measures are available.

3. *Stroop Color and Word Test.* There are a number of variations of this test. This test takes about five minutes to administer and score (Golden, 1978).

The Stroop Color and Word Test measures both mental speed and attention. The subject is required to look at a list of words printed in different color inks. The subject must name the color in which each word is printed, but ignore the meaning of the word. The words are the names of colors, so the subject must inhibit paying attention to the meaning of the words in order to accomplish this task in a speedy fashion.

The test is sensitive to disruptions of the capacity to concentrate and inhibit extraneous stimulation. Neurotoxicity can cause this type of mental disruption.

This test is available in paper and pencil form which can be administered to a group (Baehr and Corsini, 1980).

4. *Trails Test.* The Trailmaking Test has parts A and B. The test takes a few minutes to administer and score.

The Trailmaking Test was part of the Army Individual Test Battery (Lezak, 1983). It is widely used because the test is easily administered and scored, and it is very sensitive to brain dysfunction. Functions measured by this test include visuomotor tracking, psychomotor speed, and the ability to rapidly change attention. Part B requires the subject to rapidly connect a series of circles, while alternating numbers and letters (Figure 3-4). Practice effects were not evident upon repeated testing (Lezak, 1982).

5. *Grooved Pegboard Test* (Lezak, 1983). This test measures manual dexterity. It used a pegboard with slotted holes, and pegs that fit in the holes in only

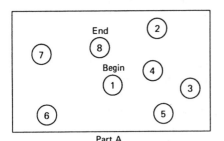

Part A

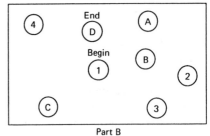

Part B

Figure 3-4. Sample of the Trail Making Test. From Lezak, M.D. 1983. *Neuropsychological Assessment.* New York: Oxford University Press. Reproduced with permission.

one orientation. The subject picks up the pegs as rapidly as possible, and places the pegs in the slotted peg holes. Manual dexterity may be depressed by peripheral nerve dysfunction, affecting sensory or motor control of the fingers. It is not a very sensitive test of neurotoxicity, but it adapts well for repeated measurements; it is easy to administer and score, and subjects find the test easy to take.

6. *Benton Visual Retention Test* (Benton, 1974). This test measures the ability to remember complex visual figures and reproduce them when the stimulus is removed. See Figure 3-5 for an example of the types of designs presented.

Three equivalent forms are available. The test takes about five minutes to administer. Scoring is somewhat involved, and requires a thorough study of the manual. However, this test is sensitive to neurotoxicity, and it deserves consideration even though it is more difficult to score than other tests.

When given without the benefit of baseline measures, this test is still useful, as the norms include specifications for age and estimated pre-exposure ability. Repeated measurement should not pose a problem; Lezak (1982) found that three administrations, given to normal control subjects six and twelve months apart, produced no significant differences.

7. *Paced Auditory Serial Addition Test* (PASAT) (Lezak, 1983). This test measures mental tracking, attention, and mental fluidity. It is relatively difficult to understand, and may not be useful when testing individuals with low average intelligence. However, it may be very useful if the workers are above average intelligence.

The test requires the subject to listen to a long string of numbers, which are

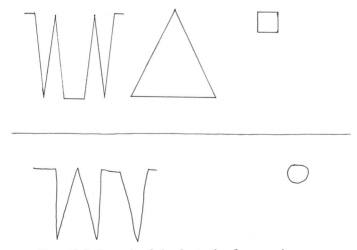

Figure 3-5. Example of visual retention figures and responses.

read at a rate of about one every two seconds. Consecutive numbers are added. The task is difficult, because the need to perform the addition interferes with hearing the next number, and remembering the previous number. For example, if the list of numbers includes 3 − 4 − 6 − 1, the subject replies 7 after hearing the number 4, 10 after hearing the number 6, and 7 after hearing the number 1. The numbers are usually presented using a tape recorder. This test could also be given to a group, with the subjects writing the numbers. However, the results may be different from the results of the standard administration.

8. *Vocabulary Test.* Vocabulary is resistant to the effects of neurotoxicity. It can be measured with a number of tests, including a subject of the WAIS-R (Wechsler, 1981). Vocabulary should be assessed at baseline (pre-employment), but is can also be used as a relative ''anchor'' to assess possible changes in brain functions that are more susceptible to neurotoxicity.

Vocabulary level reflects a person's general intellectual ability, and has been used by neuropsychologists to determine pre-sickness mental ability. Its robustness even in the presence of diffuse brains damage has been demonstrated (Lezak, 1983). Interpretation of this test must take educational level into account.

Using the WAIS-R, vocabulary is assessed by having the subject define a list of words. The answers are recorded and scored on a two point scale. Vocabulary can also be assessed in group situations with multiple-choice type vocabulary tests, and such tests have been devised for nonverbal responses.

9. *Malingering.* A number of tests are available to assess malingering (Singer, 1988c), but this type of evaluation may be better accomplished after a worker is selected for further testing.

10. *Block Design Test.* This test requires the subject to reproduce a two-dimensional design using colored blocks. The most common example of this test can be found in Wechsler (1981). The Block Design Test measures the constructional function. Although this test is often sensitive to neurotoxicity, because Wechsler (1981) does not offer equivalent versions for repeated testing, it may not be suitable for repeated measures.

Repeated Measurement. With repeated measurements, some improvement in function may be found as the subject learns how to perform the task. Practically speaking, if the subject can retain this information over a six to twelve month period, the subject probably has not been severely affected by exposure. To avoid this problem, the testing can be given repeatedly every other day for a week until a baseline performance level is established, but this precaution seems to be unnecessary.

Some of the measures recommended above are part of the Repeatable Cognitive Perceptual Battery (Lewis and Rennick, 1979). In their studies of the battery, practice effects did not pose a problem. Lewis et al. (1989) presented a normative study of the battery, which may be useful if workers are tested post-employment, and baseline testing was not done.

In general with psychometric or biologic testing, comparison of repeated psychometric tests would be more reliable if the testing is done on the same day of the week and close to the same day of the week and close to the same time of day. There are daily rhythms that affect all people which may affect test performance. In any case, if an abnormality is found, the subject should be retested. If the abnormality persists, then the subject can be referred for further examination.

Neurophysiologic Tests

Neurophysiologic tests can also be used to evaluate neurotoxicity. The tests selected should be portable and easy for technicians to administer. The equipment should be robust in terms of relative lack of interference from extraneous electrical sources. Portability is advisable. The results should be valid and reliable. See the previous section in this chapter on the criteria of test selection.

Nerve Conduction Velocity Testing.   Nerve conduction velocity (NCV) testing has been widely used in the evaluation of occupational and environmental toxicity. Figure 3-6 shows an example of NCV equipment. NCV measures the

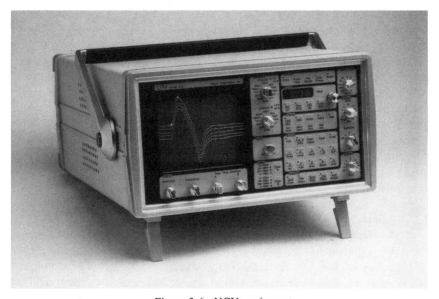

Figure 3-6. NCV equipment.

time it takes for nerve impulses to travel in the arms and legs. NCV has been applied to the epidemiologic assessment of neurotoxicity of exposure to lead and arsenic (Singer, in press); mercury (Singer et al., 1987); lead (Singer et al. 1983); herbicides (Singer et al., 1982); and many other substances by many other researchers. For overall descriptions of the technique, see Kimura (1983) and Ma and Liveson (1983). See Chapter 2 for a description of the technique.

The sensitivity of NCV for the evaluation of neurotoxicity depends upon:

1. *Selection of nerves for measurement: Location of nerve segments.* Nerve fibers in the arms and feet are more sensitive to many types of toxicity than nerve fibers located closer to the spine. Normal maintenance of the nerve pathway can be disrupted by toxic agents. The center of nerve nutrition is located in the spine. The farther a nerve fiber is from its source of nutrition, the more sensitive it is to disruption of its vital processes.

2. *Selection of nerves for measurement. Sensory versus motor nerves.* Reduction in sensory NCV and amplitude appears to be more prevalent than reduction in motor NCV or amplitude with many types of toxicity, suggesting that in general, sensory nerve fibers are more vulnerable to neurotoxicity than are motor fibers.

3. *Nerve temperature.* NCV is reduced by about 2.4 meters per second per degree centigrade (Kimura, 1983). Temperature can be controlled by electric heating pads applied to the limb being tested. However, the temperature of the limb must be measured to insure accurate results. This value can then be used to adjust the NCV to a standard temperature. Because of the linear correlation between skin and subcutaneous temperature, surface electrodes can be used to evaluate temperature (Kimura, 1983).

4. *Age.* Statistically speaking, NCV decreases about 2 meters per second per decade in adults. This may not present a problem when NCV is assessed every six to twelve months, and can, in any event, be accounted for in the statistical treatment of the difference scores.

5. *Bilateral assessment.* NCV should be assessed on both limbs when screening for neurotoxicity. Positive findings in both limbs would suggest the need for further investigation. Bilateral assessment will reduce the possibility of false positive identification. There is little reason why neurotoxic agents would affect one limb and not the other, while an injury or compression of a nerve may affect only one limb. Both limbs should be assessed to determine if neurotoxicity is present.

6. *Statistical treatment of the data.* When data is pooled, the sensitivity of the test is increased. This topic is discussed below.

7. *Technical training.* The technician who measures NCV will need to learn the sites to which the electrodes should be applied, and other matters. The sensitivity of the technique will depend upon reliable and valid data gathering procedures. A nurse could be trained for this task.

Sural NCV Measurement. The sural nerve, from the calf to the ankle, is a good choice for neurotoxicity screening. It appears to be vulnerable to many neurotoxic substances, and for that reason has been used for many research studies. (See Singer (in press); Singer et al. (1987); Singer et al. (1983); and Singer et al. (1982).) Many other studies have examined sural NCV response to neurotoxic agents.

Limb preparation for this measurement takes a few minutes. Some time may be necessary to warm the limb in cold climatic conditions. The warming can be accomplished with heating pads or infrared lamps. The actual measurement usually takes just a few minutes. However, if the leg has a thick fat layer, or if the nerve is deteriorated, the NCV may take more time to be measured.

Other Types of Nerve Conduction Studies. Techniques of repetitive stimulation and computer analysis of the nerve evoked potential waveform may be helpful in neurotoxicity screening programs.

Cortical Evoked Potential. Somatosensory and auditory evoked potential measurement, and endogenously generate cortical potentials, may be used in neurotoxicity screening. See Chapter 2 for a discussion of this approach.

DATA ANALYSIS

In addition to individual analysis, neurotoxicity screening data should be analyzed as a group. By pooling data over the group, small changes that may be significant can more easily be detected.

The detection of neurotoxic effects can be viewed from the "signal detection" perspective. Signal detection describes a method of information processing. In order to detect a signal, the important information must be extracted from random information (noise).

Random alterations of neural function can mask true neurotoxic deterioration. By using statistical analysis, the random fluctuations are mathematically controlled. If a score (individual or group averaged value) fluctuates beyond what would be expected by chance alone, then chance is not likely to be the cause of the fluctuation. When performing neurotoxicity screening, the cause of the fluctuation may well be neurotoxicity.

Statistics. For examples of the statistical handling of neuro-epidemiologic data see Singer (in press); Singer at al. (1987); Valciukas et al. (1985); Singer et al. (1983); Singer et al. (1982); Valciukas and Singer (1982); and Valciukas et al. (1980).

Basic statistical treatment of data would include the calculation of the average score, often called the mean. In neurotoxicity screening the subject will have measurements taken over a period of time. A difference score can be calculated by subtracting the value taken at a later time from the baseline value. The difference scores across people can be averaged. This mean difference score is then divided by the expected fluctuation of the scores. The resulting number is located on the bell-shaped curve which models the normal distribution of biological data. If the location is at the extremes of the curve, then an abnormality has been detected.

This procedure may sound complicated, but it has been used to analyze scientific data for about 100 years. Many biomedical, agricultural, and social scientific enterprises would halt if statistical data treatment were not utilized. It has a long history of effective use, and can easily be applied to neurotoxicity screening programs.

FOLLOWUP

Positive Results in a Group.   If neurotoxicity screening identifies neurologic decrements in a group, industrial hygiene and safety engineers should be consulted to determine the cause. Suitable investigations can then be conducted to identify the possible neurotoxic chemical exposures.

Positive Results in an Individual.   Further testing should be instituted to rule out other possible causes of the neurologic decrement. A physician or neuropsychologist could interview the subject to determine the need for further testing. If such testing is indicated, a complete neuropsychological testing procedure could be administered. This would consist of tests described earlier in this chapter. If the tests are positive, the doctor can assist in the design of a treatment plan, and recommend referrals to other health professionals. Specialists may have to be consulted to rule out other possible causes of the illness, and to treat acute illness.

Treatment.   The first line of treatment is the identification of possible exposures to neurotoxic agents, at work or at home, or both. The cause of the dysfunction may be domestic exposures to chemicals, such as termite or cockroach insecticides.

Neurotoxically-affected people often require the care of a neuropsychologist who understands the ramifications of neurotoxic brain disease. Emotional difficulties often cause extreme strains on family relationships and other social interactions. Cognitive dysfunction causes problems with everyday memory and concentration. These conditions can be helped by appropriate counselling or retraining. A number of specialized cognitive retraining programs are available. The suitability of these programs for an individual affected by neurotoxicity should be carefully evaluated.

With heavy metal poisoning, some doctors recommend chelation treatment.

This therapy involves the administration of a drug that attracts and binds heavy metals. The bonded metals go into the bloodstream, and are eliminated by the kidneys and other organs of elimination. The safety of this procedure is still not certain. Perhaps it is safer for the metals to remain in place, and be gradually eliminated as the cells holding the metals break down.

General Hygienic Measures

Nutrition. Nutrition is extremely important for day-to-day health. Without proper nutrition, body cells cannot be optimally regenerated. Various diseases have been attributed to improper diet, including heart disease, cancer, and skin disorders.

Although controversy about proper nutrition exists, in general, the modern trend is towards more natural food selection and preparation. Dietary fat, excessive salt, and sugar are discouraged, and whole grains and vegetables are encouraged.

Exercise. Exercise is important for people who suffer from neurotoxicity. Pain and fatigue from neurotoxicity, and social difficulties caused by impaired mental abilities can cause neurotoxicity patients to become increasingly weaker because of a lack of physical activity.

Neurotoxicity patients may need special training to help them maintain an exercise program. Often they cannot perform vigorous exercise which they may have been capable of before exposure. Less strenuous exercises may be appropriate.

REFERENCES

Anastasi, A. 1988. *Psychological Testing*, 6th Ed. Macmillan Publishing Company: New York.

Baehr, M. E. and Corsini, R. J. 1980. *The Press Test.* Human Resources Center, University of Chicago, Press: Park Ridge, IL.

Benton, A. L.; Hamsher, K. deS.; Varney, N. R., and Spreen, O. 1983. *Contributions to Neuropsycholgical Assessment: A Clinical Manual.* Oxford University Press: New York.

Benton, A. 1974. *Manual for the Visual Retention Test.* Psychological Corporation: New York.

Blau, T. 1984. *The Psychologist as Expert Witness.* Wiley-Interscience; New York.

Blau, T. 1989. The Neuropsychologist Goes to Court. Paper presented at the National Academy of Neuropsychology Ninth Annual Meeting, Washington, DC. Psychological Seminars, Inc.: Tampa.

Golden, C. J. 1978. *Stroop Color and Word Test.* Stoelting Company: Chicago.

Guilford, J. P. and Fruchter, B. 1978. *Fundamental Statistics in Psychology and Education.* McGraw-Hill: New York.

Kimura, J. 1983. *Electrodiagnosis in Diseases of Nerve and Muscle: Principles and Practice*. F. A. Davis: Philadelphia.

Lewis R., Kelland D. Z., and Kupke, T. 1989. A normative study of the repeatable cognitive-perceptual-motor battery. Paper presented at the National Academy of Neuropsychology Annual Meeting, November, Washington, DC.

Lewis R. F. and Rennick, P. M. 1979. *Manual for the Repeatable Cognitive-Perceptual-Motor battery*. Axon Publishing Company: Grosse Pointe Park, Michigan.

Lezak, M. D. 1983. *Neuropsychological Assessment*. Oxford: University Press, New York.

Lezak, M. D. 1982. *The test-retest stability and reliability of some tests commonly used in neuropsychological assessment*. Paper presented at the Fifth European Conference of the International Neuropsychological Society, Deauville, France. Published in Lezak (1983).

Ma, D. M. and Liveson, J. A. 1983. *Nerve Conduction Handbook*. F. A. Davis: Philadelphia.

McNemar, Q. 1969. *Psychological Statistics*. 4th Ed. Wiley: New York.

Shuman, D. W. 1986. *Psychiatric and Psychological Evidence*. McGraw-Hill: New York.

Singer, R. (in press, 1990) Nervous system monitoring for early signs of chemical toxicity. *Biological Monitoring of Exposure to Metals*. John Wiley & Sons: New York.

Singer, R. 1988a. Early recognition of toxicity by assessing nervous system function. *Biomedical and Environmental Sciences*, 1: 365-362.

Singer, R. 1988b, March. *Neurotoxicity reduction*. Testimony to the United States Public Health Service, Regional Hearings on National Health Objectives for the Year 2000: New York.

Singer, R. 1988c, December. *Neurotoxicity or Nothing?: Deficit Measurement and Malingering*. Paper presented at the Third International Symposium on Neurobehavioral Methods in Occupational and Environmental Health, World Health Organization: Washington D.C.

Singer, R. 1986a. Future directions of toxicology: A neurotoxicologist's point of view. *Journal of the American College of Toxicology*, 5(6): 603.

Singer, R. 1986b. Managing the risk of occupational toxicity. *Journal of the American College of Toxicology*, 5(6): 603.

Singer, R. 1986c. Prevention of neurotoxicity at the workplace. *The Toxicologist*, 6(1): 283.

Singer, R. 1985a. A model neurotoxicity prevention program for biological monitoring of workers at risk. *Journal of the American College of Toxicology*. 4(6): 348.

Singer, R. 1985b, September. *Prevention of neurotoxicity*. Testimony presented to the United States Food and Drug Administration Symposium on Predicting Neurotoxicity from Preclinical Data. Washington, D.C.

Singer, R.; Valciukas, J. and Rosenman, K. D. 1987. Peripheral neurotoxicity in workers exposed to inorganic mercury compounds. *Archives of Environmental Health*, 42(4): 181-184.

Singer, R.; Valciukas, J. and Lilis, R. 1983. Lead exposure and nerve conduction velocity: The differential time course of sensory and motor nerve effects. *Neurotoxicology*, 4(2): 193-202.

Singer, R.; Moses, M.; Valciukas, J.; Lilis, R. and Selikoff, I. J. 1982. Nerve conduction velocity studies of workers employed in the manufacture of phenoxy herbicides. *Environmental Research* 29: 297–311.

Smith, A. 1973. *Symbol Digits Modality Test*. Western Psychological Services: Los Angeles.

Valciukas, J.; Lilis, R.; Singer, R.; Glickman, L. and Nicholson, W. J. 1985. Neurobehavioral changes among shipyard painters exposed to solvents. *Archives of Environmental Health*, 40(1): 47–52.

Valciukas, J. and Singer, R. 1982. The embedded figures test in epidemiological studies of environmental neurotoxic agents. *Environmental Research*, 28: 183–198.

Valciukas, J.; Lilis, R.; Singer, R.; Fischbein, A.; Anderson, H. A., and Glickman, L. 1980. Lead exposure and behavioral changes: Comparisons of three occupational groups with different levels of lead absorption. *American Journal of Industrial Medicine*, 1: 421–462.

Wechsler, D. 1981. *WAIS-R Manual*. Psychological Corporation: New York.

4

FORENSIC ASPECTS OF NEUROTOXICITY

CORPORATE AND MANAGERIAL REASONS FOR CONCERNS
ABOUT NEUROTOXICITY

Legal. When potentially harmful products are produced, an injury may result. An affected party may sue. Lawsuits immediately come to mind when discussing the types of societal problems that may arise because of industrial production of potentially hazardous products. This is an unfortunate aspect of our societal structure, for a number of reasons.

1. The resolution of the problem usually occurs after the disease process and the resultant pain and suffering. Even if a monetary reward passes to the plaintiff, there is no adequate compensation for loss of good health.

2. The legal system is based upon an adversarial process, where parties contest the truthfulness of a claim; it is not based upon a system of cooperation. Thus the adversarial process often leads to effort and energy expended solely for the promotion of individual gain, rather than to cooperation which promotes the common welfare.

3. Our legal system promotes the concept of scarcity and guilt. These concepts are detrimental to mental health. Scarcity arouses feelings of insecurity and hopelessness, while guilt creates attempts by the accused to deny mistakes of the past and a refusal to help, at times, when help is needed. In criminal proceedings, guilt is so emphasized that the accused only has two options: guilty or not guilty. The possibility of innocence is not part of the judgement.

4. Legal proceedings are wasteful of money, time, and energy. Money is transferred to lawyers who actually are third parties and not directly involved in the relationship between the plaintiff and the defendant. The plaintiff's attorney's fee is often one-third of the sum awarded to the plaintiff, while the defendant's attorney accumulate weeks or months of hourly fees at rates often above $150 per hour. Defense attorneys are trained to try and out spend the plaintiff (who usually has fewer financial resources than the corporation being sued) in order to financially and psychologically exhaust the plaintiff before the trial. Defense attorneys often drag out judicial proceedings, with minimally justifiable legal maneuvers to further obfuscate the issues at hand.

5. Criminal proceedings are becoming more frequent as corporate executives are being prosecuted for negligence and environmental pollution.

Public Relations.   Adverse publicity decreases sales. If products are marketed without adequate safeguards, by the laws of probability, people are bound to be injured. People are now suspicious of chemical products. If injuries occur from a product, word of the dangerous nature of the product spreads, and people become wary about purchasing the product. Profits can plummet. In the long run, a company's best interest is the production of articles which are in the customer's best interest, with adequate safeguards and warnings against hazardous properties.

Poor Employee Relations.   If an employee becomes sick from the actions of an employer, the remaining employees will begin to lose trust in the employer. A reduction of trust can cause loss of productivity.

CIVIL SUITS

The legal system can be divided into criminal and civil law. Criminal cases involve a breach of law, such as murder, theft, and spying, which offends society as a whole. Civil cases involve suits brought by one or more parties against other parties.

Legal cases involving toxic chemicals are called toxic torts. The potential liability in toxic torts is very large. The best known example is asbestos litigation, involving many thousands of plaintiffs across the country. Even when being removed, asbestos can trigger litigation. The U.S. EPA sued the New York City Board of Education for removing asbestos without proper notification. EPA was concerned that the removal may have been improperly done, leading to greater air pollution (Tolchin, 1989). In another example illustrating the size and complexity of modern toxic torts, New York City is suing five major paint manufacturers and their trade associations for more than $50 million for the costs of reducing health hazards caused by lead paint in city houses and apartment buildings (BNA, 1989a).

Asbestos litigation has been swamping state judicial dockets. In Maryland, an asbestos case filed in 1989 cannot get a trial date before 1997. Plaintiffs are filing new cases at the rate of 2,500 per year (Labaton, 1989). Asbestos is only one of many toxic hazards in our environment. It has received much publicity, in part because of the pioneering research of Dr. Irving Selikoff, founder of the Environmental Sciences Laboratory, Mt. Sinai School of Medicine. Attention paid to other environmental toxic hazards is now increasing. Will neurotoxic suits one day swamp state judicial dockets? Neurotoxic substances are certainly distributed as widely as asbestos.

Although the settlement is being contested, Union Carbide has agreed to pay $470 million in connection with the 2,500 people killed in the Bhopal, India accidental release of toxic chemicals. The substance released was methyl isocyanate, which is neurotoxic. An employee neurotoxicity monitoring program can alert or sensitize management about the possibly extreme health hazards of a product being manufactured.

Indoor pollution is an increasing cause of lawsuits. Only about a dozen such suits have been filed in the past two years, but the U.S. EPA estimated that the cost of indoor air pollution totals tens of billions of dollars annually in lost productivity, direct medical care, lost earnings, and employee sick time. According to a *Wall Street Journal* article "As scientists hone their ability to determine what levels of contamination make people sick, lawsuits are expected to grow sharply" (Marcus, 1989).

Whether one applauds or deplores the developing penchant of persons and groups to sue for toxic injuries, this tendency will probably continue. It behooves manufacturers and managers to be aware of these developments, so that they can prevent unfortunate legal problems.

The Evolution of Tort Law.

Tort is a French word meaning "wrong." The legal field of torts deals with people who claim to be injured or wronged in some way by others who are known as "tortfeasors." If the tortfeasors or their insurance company cannot reach an agreement with the claimants, then the claimants can file a lawsuit to pursue their claim. The claimants then become plaintiffs, and the tortfeasors become defendants (Shain, 1973).

There are three general categories of torts: (1) injuries resulting from negligence; (2) injuries caused by intentional acts; and (3) injuries caused by behavior which is so dangerous to the public that the law provides compensation without having to prove negligence or intention. The last category is known as strict or absolute liability (Shain, 1973).

Negligence. Negligence can be defined as carelessness. If ordinary and prudent care for others is not taken, and an injury results, then a negligent act has occurred, and the responsible person or persons may be called upon to compensate the victim. The standard of care may vary with the professional relationship with the plaintiff, ie., doctor, lawyer, industrial hygienist, etc. (Shain, 1973).

Negligence is legally defined as conduct "which falls below the standard established by law for the protection of others against reasonable harm." The "standard established by law" may be found in legislation or by applying the common law "reasonable person" standard. Determining whether conduct is reasonable depends upon (1) the probability that the injury could be predicted (foreseeability), and (2) the gravity of the injury versus the cost of avoiding injury (Axline, 1987).

Manufacturers, professionals, or others with special expertise in the activities they conduct are expected to exercise a higher degree of care in their respective activities than the ordinary person. At the minimum, an expert is expected to keep abreast of scientific knowledge and advances in his or her field, while manufacturers have the duty to test their product. Once risk of injury becomes known, the expert or manufacturer is not permitted to continue "business as usual," if such activities are careless or dangerous, even if others in the industry do so (Pollan, 1984).

In addition to negligence (in negligence cases), cause must be proven in court for damages to be awarded. The elements of causation that must be proven in a negligence case are (Pollan, 1984):

1. There exists a duty or standard of conduct for the protection of others against unreasonable harm.
2. The defendant failed to comply with that standard.
3. There is sufficient causal connection between the defendant's conduct and the plaintiff's injury (proximate cause) for the law to impose liability.
4. Actual loss or damage to the plaintiff has occurred.

Two types of damages are compensable—special and general. Special damages are the plaintiff's out-of-pocket expenses, including medical bills, lost earnings, and property damage. General damages are awarded for pain and suffering. Putative damages are awarded to punish the defendant if the negligence involves intentional, malicious, or gross negligence (Shain, 1973).

Intentional Torts.   Intentional torts include assault and battery, intentional infliction of emotional distress, invasion of property interests (trespassing), and nuisance (the right to a tranquil life) (Shain, 1973).

Intentional tort law is being increasingly applied to toxic torts. Battery is defined as contact which is intentionally harmful or offensive. Assault occurs when the victim becomes apprehensive that a battery will immediately occur. This cause of action has been applied to an employer on the basis that he "assaulted" an employee with toxic chemicals during the normal work situation (Axline, 1987).

Both trespassing and nuisance may apply to toxic torts. It is conceivable that legal action could be brought for trespass for the uninformed introduction into a person's body of toxic substances, and for nuisance, if the substances interfere in some way with a tranquil life. Emotional distress is a frequent element of damages in nuisance cases (Axline, 1987).

Strict or Absolute Liability.   Absolute liability occurs when an activity is so dangerous that its very performance makes an owner, operator or manufacturer strictly liable for any damages that might result. These activities have been called ultra-hazardous. Activities that have been classified as ultra-hazardous include blasting with explosives and fumigating with deadly poisons (Shain, 1973).

Strict liability is a recent common law development that is intended to induce industry to be more responsive to the public welfare by allowing recovery of damages without proving fault. A party that manufactures or sells a defective product that is unreasonably hazardous, is liable to the user or consumer. Most toxic tort actions are brought under the theory of strict liability, because proof of negligence or breach of warranty is not needed (Pollan, 1984).

In strict liability, the focus is on the condition of the product, not the conduct of the defendant. In addition to application regarding products, strict liability can also apply to toxic waste situations (Pollan, 1984).

Product Liability. Plaintiffs injured by defective products formerly recovered damages under two theories of law: breach of warranty and negligence. Strict liability can now be added to the list (Shain, 1973).

Breach of warranty occurs if the product does not perform as well as it should. Negligence occurs if a manufacturer or vendor fails to exercise reasonable care in the manufacture or design of a product, or fails to warn of dangerous properties, or fails to test, or instruct the purchaser in proper use of the product (Shain, 1973).

Strict liability eliminates the need to prove fault. It has been applied to product liability cases involving toxic substances (Axline, 1987). Strict liability was based on the idea that businesses must bear the responsibility and burden for placing defective products in the market. The injured party does not have to prove breach of warranty or negligence. Anyone who sells a product in a defective condition is liable for damages resulting from that product (Shain, 1973).

A defective condition is one that is unreasonably dangerous to consumers. Some products maybe intrinsically dangerous. If the manufacturer fails to warn of the dangers of the product, the product is legally defective, and the manufacturer is liable for the injury (Shain, 1973).

Failure to Warn. Many toxic torts alleging strict product liability are failure to warn cases (Pollan, 1984). Unreasonable conduct includes the failure to warn, or failure to adequately warn of possible injuries. Liability for failure to warn arises if the manufacturer or supplier:

1. Knows or has reason to know that the product is or is likely to be dangerous for the use for which it is supplied.
2. Has no reason to believe that those for whom the product is supplied will realize its dangerous condition.

3. Fails to exercise reasonable care to inform potential users of the product's dangerous condition or of the facts which make it likely to be dangerous.

Failure to provide adequate warning may result in liability for negligence, for breach of warranty, or for a defective or unreasonably dangerous product (Axline, 1987).

Breach of the duty to warn is probably the standard of care relied upon most frequently in toxic tort cases. It is relatively easy to warn of a product's hazardous or toxic properties. The appropriate warning can "cure" or remedy the defect in the product. Courts have found that even if the technology does not exist, or is prohibitively expensive, to eliminate the danger of a toxic agent and the toxic agent is too useful to society to prohibit its creation or use, the providing of a warning is neither impossible nor prohibitively expensive (Pollan, 1984).

The amount of care that a defendant must take increases with the risk of harm. The duty to warn arises whenever an ordinary, prudent person (or expert) would have given a warning to protect another person against foreseeable and unreasonable risk of harm. Since manufacturers and/or experts are required to keep abreast of developments in their field, they have a continuing responsibility to warn the consumers or their clients of dangers that come to their attention (Pollan, 1984).

The duty to warn is composed of two separate duties: (1) a duty to give adequate and comprehensible instructions for safe use, and (2) a duty to warn of dangers inherent in improper use. For a warning to be adequate, it must be effective. Even if a warning is adequate, its efficacy can be eroded by negligent over-promotion of the product (Pollan, 1984).

Courts may apply a strict standard when evaluating the adequacy of warnings. For example, in a New Mexico appellate court, a case was brought involving grain that was treated with seed disinfectant and fed to hogs. Children who ate meat from the hogs developed neurotoxicity. The label on the disinfectant warned it was poisonous and should not be used on feed. However, the court held that the label was not adequate to warn people that the resulting meat could be poisoned (Pollan, 1984). This reasoning may apply to other legal actions involving pesticides and food.

Employees who are notified of possible health risks on the job may lose their ability to recover damages on the grounds that they were warned of hazards they might encounter. If the workers decides to continue their work, they may appear to have assumed the risk of employment and toxic chemical exposure. However, informed consent and voluntary agreement require full disclosure of risk.

Fraudulent Misrepresentation of Concealment.   Toxic torts often contend that there is an element of fraudulent misrepresentation or concealment. If this can be proved, the stakes are raised on punitive damages, longer statutes of limitations, and avoidance of the exclusivity of worker compensation remedies (Pollan, 1984).

The New Jersey Supreme Court on May 31, 1989, upheld a 1987 jury verdict that awarded $1.4 million in compensatory and punitive damages to six current and former workers who developed disease from workplace exposure. It agreed that there was sufficient evidence to support the jury's finding that the disease was aggravated by the company and its doctor's fraudulent concealment of the worker's disabilities (Anonymous, 1989).

Potential Areas for Concern for Manufacturers of Neurotoxic Substances. Many substances are neurotoxic. The tables provided in Chapter 1 show the types of substances that are neurotoxic and the types of occupations that involve exposure to neurotoxic agents. This knowledge is available to manufacturers, who have the duty to warn workers, users, and consumers of the possibility of neurotoxicity.

As people become more aware of the possibility of neurotoxicity, lawsuits will increase. The potential liability of manufacturers of neurotoxic substances is enormous. Suppose relatives of Alzheimer patients believe that the disease was caused by a particular substance or group of products. Class action suits regarding Alzheimer's disease seems like a remote nightmare, but possibly they could occur. People who work with neurotoxic substances and develop neurological disease could also form class action suits. Appropriate warnings may reduce the liability of manufacturers and distributors.

In addition to civil suits, criminal sanctions for injuries due to toxic products and manufacturing procedures are being applied to managers. This will be described below.

Potential Areas for Concern for Professionals and Manufacturers of Neurotoxic Substances. Experts, industrial hygienists, safety engineers, and other personnel have a duty to stay abreast of their field, and to be aware of the potential neurotoxicity of substances for which they are responsible. They also have the duty to warn their employers or clients of possible neurotoxic hazards. Failure to complete these duties may put the professional at risk of a suit from their employer or client. In addition, criminal sanctions for toxic injury are being applied to negligent managers.

It may even be possible to sue government agencies and employees for damages resulting from failure to set standards, deviation from mandated procedure, or failure to perform what is a clear duty under federal law. The U.S. Supreme Court ruled that such claims may be barred only if the conduct involves the permissible exercise of policy judgement (Anonymous, 1988).

Recently, The American Chemical Society has announced an insurance plan to protect members from liability claims from professional activities. This shows the concern of members for such suits (Schreiner, 1989).

WORKER'S COMPENSATION

Lawsuits for injuries occurring at the workplace usually are held in Worker's Compensation Hearings. These legal proceedings were formerly the exclusive court for injuries at the workplace. However, workers are finding ways to bring suits in civil court, with the expectation of greater compensation. Some states allow willful action or misconduct as grounds for a civil suit. In Ohio, if an employer knew that an employee was being exposed to toxic chemicals, and failed to correct the situation or warn the employee, a cause for action for an intentional tort in civil court may exist. In several states, if an employer fails to inform an employee of the existence of a disease caused by exposure to toxic substances in the workplace, the employee may bypass the workers compensation system and sue the employer directly for aggravation of symptoms (Barnard, 1984).

In a recent New Jersey case, workers compensation laws did not prevent an employee from suing his employer with a claim that the employer aggravated an on-the-job injury. Workers may sue employers who conceal knowledge that their jobs have caused them disease, according to the New Jersey Supreme Court. The ruling overturned a lower court decision that held that a company was protected from lawsuits because it already paid claims through the state workers compensation law (Anonymous, 1986). Concealing knowledge of an injury or disease may also involve criminal sanctions. In Connecticut, a bill was recently passed to allow workers who have been exposed to toxic substances in the workplace to sue their employers (CLT, 1989). Third party suits are also available to workers, allow injured worker to sue the manufacturer of toxic substances in civil court.

CRIMINAL LIABILITY FOR TOXIC INJURY

A new trend has arisen in our legal system. Under certain circumstances, managers of corporations and other employers are being tried for criminal charges if workers are injured. A notable instance occurred in 1985, when a former company president, a plant supervisor, and a foreman were each sentenced to 25 years in prison, and fined $10,000, for involuntary manslaughter and reckless conduct (Burnett, 1985).

In the last few years, prosecutors in many states have brought hundreds of criminal cases against employers for safety violations. However, there has been some concern whether states actually have these rights (Greenhouse, 1989).

The U.S. Supreme Court has recently permitted such prosecutions to take place. A Chicago manufacturing concern and five of its top officials were indicted on state charges of aggravated battery and reckless conduct. The indictment charged that the company, which makes coated wire, failed to provide necessary safety equipment, and repeatedly exposed its workers to dangerous substances, including polyvinyl chloride, toluene, phenol, and aluminum and copper dust. In the state court, the company argued that the prosecution had been pre-empted by federal OSHA regulations. The state supreme court did not agree, and the U.S. Supreme Court refused to hear the case (Greenhouse, 1989).

In another example of such criminal charges, the owner of a defunct battery plant pleaded guilty and received a $2\frac{1}{2}$ year sentence in federal prison for lying about dangerous lead exposure to his workers and lying about the quality of batteries he sold to the U.S. Defense Department (BNA, 1989a).

In *U.S.* v. *Protex Industries, Inc.*, CA 10, No. 88-1371, 5/11/89, a company was fined $7.6 million in a U.S. District Court, under the "knowing endangerment" provision of the Resource Conservation and Recovery Act (RCRA). Protex had exposed its employees to hazardous chemicals at a drum recycling facility (Anonymous, 1989b). According to the Court, Protex showed a "callousness toward the severe physical effect prolonged exposure to toxic chemicals may cause or has caused" its workers. The U.S. prosecutor stated that the actual injury was solvent poisoning, which resulted in psycho-organic syndrome.

Psycho-organic syndrome is another term for neurotoxicity. This term has been applied particularly to solvent exposed patients. The ruling cited above illustrates the need for employers to actively take charge of potential liabilities. Neurotoxicity monitoring programs would help to control this type of liability and the danger of exposure to criminal sanctions.

The *Protex* case was analyzed by Willmore (1989), who pointed out that the decision in *Protex* involved a relatively new provision of the federal Resource Conservation and Recovery Act (RCRA; 42 U.S.C. 6928(e)), dubbed the "knowing endangerment provision." Under that provision, it is a separate federal crime to violate any of the provisions of the law regarding hazardous waste, if one knows at the time of the violation that one is placing a person in imminent danger of death or serious bodily injury. Fines of up to one million dollars and imprisonment for up to 15 years can apply. Protex argued that "psycho-organic syndrome" (neurotoxicity) did not constitute "serious bodily injury" within the meaning of the statute. However, the Court of Appeals flatly rejected this argument, and accused the company of "callousness" for having proffered this argument.

Ignorance of the law is no excuse, as affirmed by a U.S. Federal appeals court, which found that proof of knowledge of the occurrence of a toxic violation was not necessary to convict the director of a public sewage treatment system of illegal waste disposal (BNA, 1989b).

The U.S. House bill HR 2664: Corporate Criminal Liability Act, proposed penalties for managers who discover "serious concealed danger" and fail to report such danger to the appropriate federal authority. This bill was planned to be introduced in 1989 (Schreiner, 1989).

There is grass-roots support for corporate responsibility for toxic chemicals. The pension funds of New York City and of the state of California and other investors joined environmental groups and religious organizations in formulating a code of conduct to judge which corporations are environmentally responsible. The institutions which are involved control more than $100 billion (Feder, 1989). This creates a responsive capital market for more responsible companies.

Will state and local prosecutors continue to pursue corporate crime? The public's attitudes about corporate behavior affects the prosecutors' willingness to pursue corporate crime (Hans and Erman, 1989). It seems that the public is increasingly concerned about corporate crime, particularly crimes involving toxic substances.

Does the public hold corporations accountable for their behavior? The answer seems to be increasingly, yes. Support for even higher standards of responsibility to be applied to corporations is found in a study of the public's attitudes. The study was designed to determine whether people responded differently to corporate and to individual wrongdoing. The researchers found that for identical actions, the corporations were judged to be more reckless and morally responsible than individuals, and that jurors would be more willing to penalize corporations (in contrast with accused individuals) with civil and criminal penalties (Hans and Erman, 1989).

There are other indications that the public wants to get tough with corporate criminals. In November 1989, the U.S. Sentencing Commission proposed a great increase in the penalties for criminal convictions of corporations, including imposing far higher fines (fines that would at least double the penalty resulting from a crime, after paying victims full restitution) (Strasser, 1989).

In an interesting legal case involving neurotoxicity, an accused murderer was acquitted on the basis of insanity caused by neurotoxicity. The defendant claimed that radiation from uranium mines near his home caused him to go insane. According to the defendant's expert witness, "If toxins lead to brain damage, victims could become human time bombs. Even minimal brain damage makes a person much more sensitive to drugs and alcohol and is likely to result in dysfunction" (Lucas, 1989).

IS IGNORANCE BLISS?

Attorney Frances Miller, Professor of Law at Boston University's School of Law, published a 40 page article entitled "Biological Monitoring: The Employer's Dilemma," in the *American Journal of Law and Medicine* (Miller,

1984). (As described in Chapter 2, neurotoxicity monitoring is a subset of biological monitoring (BM).) BM is designed to provide the earliest and most accurate predictor of chemical toxicity at the workplace. Dr. Miller raised the question of the employer's dilemma, as follows, ''When health-conscious employers monitor the physical well-being of their employees in an effort to avoid the terrible personal and economic costs that these hazards can produce, they may be supplying their employees with the documentation necessary to recover financially for their industrial illnesses.''

Employer incentives to institute toxicity monitoring programs include:

1. Controlling occupational health costs.
2. Higher productivity because of better health and fewer accidents.
3. Fewer worker compensation and disability claims because of better health.
4. Lower health insurance premiums because of the reduced need for medical services throughout the careers of workers lifetime.
5. More harmonious relations with labor, and lower wage demands because the work is perceived as less hazardous.
6. Reduced government intervention and standard setting.
7. Fewer chances of toxic torts. Since toxicity monitoring programs are available, failure to use these programs may be evidence of willful and deliberate attempt to harm. This principle applies even if an entire industry does not comply.
8. Greater control of insurance coverage and statute of limitations problems.
   a. Insurance policies may not cover diseases that are discovered years after employment. Such a situation often occurs with toxic disease. The former employer would then have to pay.
   b. The statute of limitations for toxic disease is shifting in favor of a more liberal or scientifically based approach. This will increase insurance coverage problems.
9. Insulation of the corporate image and society from the effects of occupational illness.

Employer disincentives to implementing toxicity monitoring include:

1. Disabled employees can use monitoring information as evidence of work-related illness.
2. False positive results may lead to premature dismissal, while false negative results may permit an affected employee to remain on the job.
3. The discovery of hazardous conditions could lead unions to press for greater safety protection.
4. Monitoring techniques could have a negative health effect (ie., x-rays, tissue sampling).

5. Results may invite government regulation, if hazards are found.
6. Management may prefer a turnover of workers to reduce the hazard to any particular worker.

After careful review of the total picture, Professor Miller concluded:

". . . employers are best served by voluntarily implementing monitoring programs where the techniques have a reasonably established predictive value, and informing employees of the results. This action eliminates the potential for tort liability, thereby confining recovery to worker compensation schedules. Although it may supply employees with evidence of causation, such evidence is likely to be discovered in the long run anyway. In the meantime, information will be generated which can help prevent the exacerbation of illness and minimize liability. Both personal and economic costs can thus be avoided.

. . . Employees, once fully informed about monitoring results and their implications, can be left to decide whether or not they wish to remain in a working environment predicted to be hazardous to their health. Although they cannot lose their worker compensation rights, such employees may be held to have assumed the risk of industrial illness for the purposes of tort litigation."

Professor Miller presented the carefully reasoned argument that it is the best interest of all parties, including management, to monitor workers for the earliest signs of toxicity. Ignorance of toxicity in the workplace is not expected to lead to a favorable outcome.

FORENSIC EVALUATION OF SINGLE CASES OF NEUROTOXICITY

Diagnosis of neurotoxicity relies heavily on the neuropsychological examination. Examples of neurotoxicity examinations and reports are presented in Chapter 5. For a comprehensive discussion of neurotoxicity examinations within the legal context, see Singer (1988a; 1988b; 1987; 1985a). For further examples of the neuropsychological examination for neurotoxicity, see Singer and Scott (1987a); Singer (in press (a); in press (b); 1985b; Singer and Scott, 1987b).

REFERENCES

Anonymous. 1989. New Jersey court upholds $1.4 million verdict against Dupont for fraudulent concealment. *Toxics Law Reporter*, 4(2):42. June 14, 1989.

Anonymous. 1989b. Protex should lead to more prosecution, DOJ attorney says; company seeks rehearing. *Toxics Law Reporter*, 4(1):14. June 7, 1989.

Anonymous. 1988. High court allows more room for suing federal regulators. *The Nation's Health*, July, 1988. p. 1.

Anonymous. 1986. N.J. court says worker may sue. *Occupat. Heal. & Safety News.* 2(2):16.

Axline, Michael. 1987. Theories of liability. In *A Guide to Toxic Torts*, edited by Margie Tyler Searcy. Matthew Bender: New York.

Barnard, Thomas H. 1984. Remedies. In *Toxic Torts: Litigation of Hazardous Cases.* Edited by G. Z. Nothstein. Shepard's/McGraw-Hill: Colorado Springs.

BNA. 1989a. New York City sues lead pigment producers, seeks at least $50 million plus punitives. *Toxics Law Reporter*, June 14, 1989. pp. 30-1.

BNA. 1989a. Battery company, president convicted of felonies over lead-contaminated waste. *Toxics Law Reporter*, July 26, 1989. pp. 214-15. Bureau of National Affairs: Washington, D.C.

BNA. 1989b. Ninth circuit affirms RCRA conviction, says knowledge of violation not required. *Toxics Law Reporter*, July 26, 1989. pp. 212-13. Bureau of National Affairs: Washington, D.C.

Burnett, John. 1985. Corporate murder verdict may not become trend, say legal experts. *Occup. Heal. & Safety*, October 1985. p. 22-59.

CLT. 1989. Right to sue. *Conn. Law Tribune*, 15(41):8. October 16, 1989.

Feder, Barnaby J. 1989. Group sets corporate code on environmental conduct. *New York Times*, September 8, 1989. p. D1.

Greenhouse, Linda. 1989. Court refuses to hear occupational safety appeal. *New York Times*. October 3, 1989. p. A17.

Hans, Valerie P. and Ermann, M. David. 1989. Responses to corporate versus individual wrongdoing. *Law and Human Behavior*, 13(2):151-63.

Labaton, Stephen. 1989. Manville's trust for asbestos victims runs low. *New York Times*. October 24, 1989. p. A18.

Lucas, Charlotte A. 1989. ''Toxin defense'' successful. *National Law Journal*, May 1, 1989. p. 9.

Marcus, Amy D. 1989. In some workplaces, ill winds blow. *Wall Street Journal*, October 9, 1989. p. B1.

Miller, Frances. 1984. Biological monitoring: The employer's dilemma. *American Journal of Law and Medicine* 9(1):387-426.

Pollan, Lynne. 1984. Theories of liability. In *Toxic Torts: Litigation of Hazardous Cases.* Edited by G. Z. Nothstein. Shepard's/McGraw-Hill: Colorado Springs.

Rosen, Bruce S. 1986. N.J. court adopts ''Dual injury'' rule. *National Law Journal*, December 30, 1989. p. 3.

Schreiner, Ceinwen A. 1989. For your information: Professional liability. *American College of Toxicology Newsletter*. September, 1989.

Shain, Henry. 1973. *Legal First Aid*. Funk & Wagnalls: New York.

Singer, R. (In press (a)). Neurotoxicity can produce ''MS-like'' symptoms. *Journal of Clinical and Experimental Neuropsychology*.

Singer, R. (In press (b)). Formaldehyde neurotoxicity. *Archives of Clinical Neuropsychology*.

Singer, R. 1988a. Methodology of forensic neurotoxicity evaluation: PCB case. *Toxicology*, 49:403-408.

Singer, R. 1988b. *Neurotoxicity or nothing?: Deficit measurement and malingering*. Paper presented at the Third International Symposium on Neurohehavioral Methods in Occupational and Environmental Health, World Health Organization: Washington D.C.

Singer, R. 1987. How to prove nervous system dysfunction. *A Guide to Toxic Torts*. New York: Matthew Bender.

Singer, R. 1985a. Proving damages in toxic torts: Nervous system dysfunction. *TRIAL*, November, 1985. pp. 59–60.

Singer, R. 1985b. Neuropsychological evaluation of neurotoxicity. In *Neurobehavioural Methods in Occupational and Environmental Health: Document 3. Environmental Health*. pp. 86–90. Second International Symposium, Copenhagen, Denmark: World Health Organization Regional Office for Europe.

Singer, R. and Scott, N. E. 1987a. Progression of neuropsychological deficits following toluene diisocyanate exposure. *Archives of Clinical Neuropsychology*, 2(2):135–144.

Singer, R. and Scott, N. E. 1987b. Neuropsychological evaluation of cyclodine insecticide toxicity. *The Toxicologist*, 7(1).

Strasser, Fred. 1989. Commission would up punishment. *National Law Journal*. November 20, 1989. p. 3.

Tolchin, Martin. 1989. U.S. intensifies asbestos drive, filing 13 suits. *New York Times*. p. A1.

Willmore, Robert L. 1989. RCRA provision provides new weapon against negligent hazardous waste practices. *Occupat. Heal. & Safety*, November 1989. p. 45.

5

SELECTED NEUROTOXICITY CASE REPORTS

This chapter includes neurotoxicity reports for individuals in various occupations. The reports were selected to show the types of outcomes of neurotoxicity, and to illustrate typical neuropsychological evaluations. To protect the confidentiality of the subjects, the names are fictitious. The cases presented represent the following kinds of exposure: solvents, pesticide—shipping accident, pesticide—incidental exposure, unusual psychosis from PCB exposure, paint and lead exposure, mixed chemical exposure, and a hydrogen sulfide accident. Three examples of domestic exposure to formaldehyde are also presented.

FORENSIC NEUROTOXICOLOGIC REPORT
OF
MICHAEL SMALL

Michael Small, a 29 year old male, was evaluated on January 7, 1988 for residual nervous system effects of exposure to trichloroethane and related substances.

Exposure. Mr. Small worked as a degreasing technician from February 1985 through August 1985. He was exposed to trichloroethane, acetone and other substances. The room was 12 × 24 feet and enclosed. Mr. Small reported that he felt sick (high, buzzing sensations) during the time that he worked, and that he eventually suffered from a number of psychologically debilitating symptoms, such as paranoia, excess sleeping, jumpiness and memory problems.

Initial Impression. Mr. Small appeared normally dressed and groomed, with normal facial expressions, eye contact, and without unusual mannerisms. He was oriented to time, place and person. During testing, he was found to be fairly restless. Fine motor performance was slow and deliberate.

Symptoms. Mr. Small reported that he is "jumpy and restless." He reported problems with memory, concentration and thinking clearly; he is easily distracted, and finds difficulty in planning, and understanding others; he suffers from blank spells, misplaces objects; has difficulty understanding written material; has headaches, difficulty falling asleep, drowsiness, loss of sexual interest, fatigue, anxiety, depression, irritability, and nervousness.

Psychosocial History. Mr. Small is single and lives with his parents (because of his reduced financial means).

Psychiatric Hospitalization. None reported or found in the available medical records.

Outpatient Psychological Treatment. None reported or found in available medical records, prior to exposure.

M. Med. M.D. reported on October 28, 1985, that Mr. Small has had paranoid symptomatology during the past three months. He further reported on July 24, 1986, that Mr. Small was seen on September 5, 1985, complaining of severe nervousness and described new onset phobias. He was seen on two more occasions.

L. Reiki, Ph.D., reported on May 9, 1986, that Mr. Small was seen for seven sessions of individual psychotherapy. Initial diagnosis was adjustment disorder with mixed emotional features.

Martin Berton, Ed.D., reported on September 3, 1986 that he saw Mr. Small on that date and administered a number of tests, specifically including the WAIS. He found that the client presented a pattern of generalized anxiety disorder, social withdrawal, secondary depression, tension and physical symptoms including headache.

Hospitalization. Mr. Small reported hospitalization in 1982 (hernia).

Educational Background. GED in 1979.

Employment History. Previous employment did not include significant exposure to neurotoxic agents.

Before his work was a degreasing technician, Mr. Small was employed in a machine shop for five years. He reported working six or seven days a week, and often ten hours a day. The plant went bankrupt, so he left for his next job as a degreasing technician.

Mr. Small is currently employed as a plumber's helper for a friend. He has been working for three months.

Alcohol Use. Mr. Small reported infrequent use of alcohol, limiting himself to a drink at weddings or special engagements.

General Observations

General Demeanor. Normal. Somewhat rough, direct and unsophisticated, appropriate for his background.

Posture and Gait. Normal.

Involuntary Movements. None were noticeable.

Appearance. Mr. Small was dressed casually for the examination, and appeared to be his stated age.

Orientation. Mr. Small was oriented to time, place, and the examiner's role.

Speech. Some slurring was noted. Speech delivery was somewhat rough, with occasional misuse of words or grammatical errors (possibly consistent with his educational background).

Examination

Test-taking Behavior. Mr. Small was cooperative and appeared to be giving his "best performance." The examiner did not have the impression that he was malingering.

Previous Mental Function

Academic Records. Mr. Small's grades were generally poor. School and College Ability Tests of 1972 showed percentiles: Verbal—13; Quantitative—47; Total—25. GED, taken in 1979 showed an average percentile rank of 45. His reading skills were at the 46th percentile.

Estimation. A pre-exposure percentile rank of 35 was estimated, corresponding with an IQ of 95, standard score of 9. A pre-exposure verbal percentile rank of 29 was estimated, corresponding to a verbal IQ of 92.

Test Results and Interpretation

Wechsler Adult Intelligence Scale, Revised: WAOS-R

	Scaled Scores Age-Adjusted	Percentile Rank
Verbal Subscales		
Information	6	9
Digit Span	4	2*
Vocabulary	7	16
Arithmetic	6	9*
Comprehension	9	37
Similarities	9	37
Performance Subscales		
Picture Completion	11	63
Picture Arrangement	13	84
Block Design	10	50
Object Assembly	10	50
Digit Symbol	7	16*
Verbal IQ	80	Low Average
Performance IQ	101	Average
Full Scale IQ	87	Low Average

*Deficit

Current Mental Function

Mr. Small scored in the low average range. He showed *deficits* in Digit Span (short-term memory) and Arithmetic (quantitative skills). On Digit Span, Mr. Small was unable to reliably repeat three numbers in the backwards direction. Mr. Small scored at the 69th percentile in the mathematics section of the GED in 1979.

Mr. Small took the WAIS in 1986. At that time, he performed the Digit Symbol test at the 12 scaled score, while in 1988 his scaled score on this test was 7, a significant decline in psychomotor speed and mental flexibility.

Benton Visual Retention Test.   This test assesses recent visual memory. Based upon a pre-morbid verbal IQ of 92, 8 of 10 designs were expected to be correct, with 6 errors in reproduction. Mr. Small remembered 5 designs, with 8 errors in reproduction. This performance raises the possibility of acquired impairment of cognitive function.

Wechsler Memory Scale: Logical Memory.   Based upon Mr. Small's estimated premorbid verbal IQ of 92, it was expected that he would remember 18 elements upon immediate testing. Mr. Small remembered 14 elements of the two stories upon immediate testing, which was *deficient* ($p < 0.7$). Based upon results from immediate testing, Mr. Small was expected to remember 13 elements upon delayed testing. He remembered 8, which was *deficient* ($p < .02$).

Wechsler Memory Scale: Paired-Associate Learning Test Expanded.   This test evaluates the ability to learn and remember word pairs. The score on the immediate administration was 18 (7.3 percentile based upon age) (deficit) and on the delayed administration was 10 (43rd percentile based upon age), borderline *deficit.*

The Embedded Figures Test.   This test evaluates the ability to detect visual figure-ground relationships. Mr. Small detected 33 of the 40 objects, which is within normal range.

The Grooved Pegboard Test.   This test evaluates manual dexterity. Time for completion was 78 seconds for the dominant hand, which is approximately at the 23rd percentile, and 75 seconds for the nondominant hand, which is approximately at the 36th percentile, within low normal range.

The Trailmaking Test.   This test evaluates visuomotor tracking and attention. Time for completing Part A was 37 seconds, which is approximately at the 3rd percentile, *deficit.* Time for completing Part B was 95 seconds, which is approximately at the 1st percentile, *deficit.*

The Paced Auditory Serial Addition Test.   This test evaluates verbal fluency. Mr. Small's performance was measured at the 2nd percentile, *deficit.*

The Controlled Oral Word Association Test.   This test evaluates verbal fluency. Mr. Small's performance was measured at the 2nd percentile, *deficit.*

Test Results

Deficit.   Immediate recall, quantitative skills, psychomotor speed and mental flexibility, recent memory, delayed memory, visuomotor tracking and attention, auditory information processing and tracking, and verbal fluency.

Borderline Deficits.   Visual memory and associate memory.

Malingering Tests

Clinical Interview.   No evidence for malingering was found in the course of the interview. Mr. Small's account of this exposure and condition remained constant and did not fluctuate under questioning. His demeanor and affect were appropriate and credible.

Ungrouped Dot Counting   This test is used to assess malingering. It requires the patient to count the number of dots drawn on cards. The cards are presented in a random order; if the patient is not malingering, it takes more time to count an increasing number of dots. Malingering was not found.

Endorsement of Rare Symptoms.   Six rare symptoms were included on the symptom questionnaire, none of them were chosen by Mr. Small. Malingering was not indicated.

Minnesota Multiphasic Personality Inventory (MMPI).   This test was used to assess malingering and psychological state. Malingering was not indicated on this test.

Neurophysiological Testing

Nerve conduction velocity of the median motor, median sensory and sural nerves on both sides was performed. Nerve conduction velocity and amplitude was within the normal range.

Conclusion

Within reasonable scientific certainty, Michael Small showed neuropsychological deficits associated with exposure to workplace solvents.

FORENSIC NEUROTOXICOLOGIC REPORT
OF
JOHN BENSON

John Benson was a 44 year old male evaluated on September 22, 1988 for neurotoxicity. Mr. Benson was exposed to Thimet liquid and fumes on June 16, 1986.

Chemical Description.   Thimet, an organophosphorus pesticide, is composed primarily of phorate (83% or greater phorate pesticide).

Toxicity. Phorate has a toxicity rating of 6, the most hazardous rating given. This rating corresponds with the description "super toxic"; the probable oral *lethal* dose is "a taste (less than 7 drops)." In addition to oral toxicity, Thimet can be absorbed through the skin and mucus membranes. Organophosphorus pesticides are toxic to the nervous system. Poisoning can result in brain and nerve damage as assessed by neurobehavioral and neuropsychological testing.

Exposure. On June 16, 1986, at 3 pm, Mr. Benson was supervising the unloading of a 35 foot container-van. The dimensions of this type of van are 35 feet by 8 feet by 8 feet. It has two doors that turn completely out, located on the side of the van. It is made of metal with wood panelling.

The Thimet was contained in 5 gallon pails. When the drums were being removed, a laborer noticed that one of the drums was half empty. The pallet board on which the drums were carried was brought to rest. Mr. Benson stooped to read the label. He turned the two drums in opposite directions so that he could read the labels, because the drums were rotated so that the labels were obscured.

Mr. Benson walked back into the van to determine if there was any leakage there. He did not find much moisture on the wooden floor of the van, but he did note that he "smelled the nasty taste." He estimated that he was in the van for 3 to 5 minutes.

After finishing some paperwork, Mr. Benson washed his hands, smoked a cigarette and drank some water. He could not get rid of the "rusty, metallic" taste in his mouth.

At 4:30 pm, on the way home, Mr. Benson became nauseated, dizzy, clammy, and developed a headache. His wife reports that he was stinking with a nauseating odor. This odor remained on the bedding after Mr. Benson was brought to the hospital. The hospital threw out his clothes, He was admitted to West Jefferson Hospital Emergency Room at 7:50 pm.

Summary of Exposure Details: The exact details of how Mr. Benson became wet with the pesticides is not known. However, one of the laborers who had unloaded the leaky containers gave testimony that, "The main reason [Mr. Benson] got sick, he had to get down there and read them little numbers on it, and he had to inhale it more than we did, because we didn't have to stay around it that much. But we did smell it."

According to testimony of his wife, when Mr. Benson returned home, he gave off a chemical smell, and the smell lingered on the bedding he was in contact with at home. The staff at the Hospital noticed the strong odor, they washed Mr. Benson down, and discarded his clothing. Therefore, it is likely that Mr. Benson was exposed to pesticide liquid, vapors and/or fumes, from the environment and his clothing, from around 3 pm to sometime after 8 pm that evening.

Hospital Records. At the hospital, Dr. Stein diagnosed Mr. Benson as suffering from organophosphate poisoning with evidence of motor weakness. The records do not show if blood cholinesterase levels had been determined. Dr. F. Nloser, a neurologist, found mild muscle weakness secondary to toxic exposure. Mr. Benson reports that he does not remember events that occurred the next few days.

Discharge diagnosis June 21, 1986: organophosphate exposure, brief, persistent paresthesia and hand weakness.

Medical Reports

1. M. Talm, M.D., December 28, 1987 (neurologist). Severe headaches every two or three weeks, lasting for two days. Continued numbness in right arm, predominantly in the hand. No positive findings upon physical examination. Recommended repeat EMG, including lower extremities for possible post-toxic neuropathy. Recommended MRI and complete neuropsychological evaluation.
   a. September 30, 1986. Slowing of right median sensory conduction across the carpal tunnel; scattering of sensory evoked potential. Ulnar nerve slowing at the elbow. No lower extremities done. But distal latency of median motor nerve was normal; not really compatible with carpal tunnel syndrome due to compression.
   b. October 1, 1986. EEG—no abnormalities noted.
2. Jim Tolde, M.D., December 29, 1987. Current diagnosis includes organophosphate exposure; recurrent headaches; paraesthesia in the right forearm and hand; depression; loosening and separation of teeth from gums requiring significant dental work.
3. O. Shipper, M.D., treating psychiatrist, July 11, 1988. This patient has suffered personality changes as a result of organic impairment of the central nervous system most likely due to exposure to organophosphate (which are known neurotoxins). Felt his condition was worsening.
4. F. Nloser, M.D., neurologist, July 19, 1986. CAT scan within normal limits (WNL). July 17, 1986. EEG wnl. June 17, 1986. Mild muscle weakness secondary to toxic exposure.
5. R. Clapper, M.D., Ph.D., psychiatric evaluation. Was seen for 2 hrs 15 min. at the request of defendants law firm. Concluded that Mr. Benson, "has a lot of long-standing emotional problems . . . unhappiness with his work situation . . . various domestic difficulties . . . current financial

crises." [With the exception of the last comment, I did not find evidence of Mr. Benson's long-standing emotional problems prior to the accident. Mr. Benson stated that he was happy at his job, at home, and with his friends; his wife reported a normal family life; the additional evidence available to me corroborates Mr. Benson's view of himself.]

6. C. Royal, Ph.D., clinical psychologist, February 15, 1988. Diagnosis: dementia, organic affective syndrome, r/o organic personality syndrome, adjustment disorder.

Symptoms

Interview. During my interview of Mr. Benson, he described his main symptoms as:

1. Headaches, lasting a few hours, about three or four times a week. He described the pain as severe and debilitating. He stated that doctors had prescribed narcotics for the pain but he declined and continues to decline taking habit-forming drugs.
2. Right hand numbness.
   a. Occurs about one third of the time.
   b. Numb from thumb to little finger in a semi-circle; across the wrist; and on muscle of inner forearm.
   c. During testing, it was found that his right hand was very weak, by handshake and thumb lift.
3. Emotional problems.
   a. Depression. "I always feel depressed. It's worse at times . . . sometimes I want to crawl into a corner and stay there . . . I want to get away from people."
   b. Worry. "Will this ever end? Will I be back to the same person I was before this happened?"
   c. Family difficulties. "We used to be a pretty close family, went hunting, shrimping, fishing together . . . Now we have frequent arguments. Me and my oldest son get into screaming matches, then I want to throw him out, hurt him. Half the time I don't talk to my daughter."
   d. Amotivation. He reports little or no productive activity, other than minor child care. He does not participate in former hobbies, such as hunting, fishing, woodworking, as he lacks confidence in his skills and is afraid that he or someone else will get hurt. States that he does not have the energy to do anything, has no ambition, or "the want to do something."
   e. Taste disturbance. "I could eat steak or cardboard—it tastes the same

. . . I can taste salt and the bitterness of pepper—the rest is like nothing.''

4. Difficulty reading.
5. Reduced sexual interest.

Neurotoxicity Symptom Questionnaire.   Mr. Benson endorsed many symptoms related to the nervous system. When compared to his health before the exposure, Mr. Benson found the presence of, or worsening of, symptoms including: problems with memory, concentration, attention span, thinking clearly, trouble starting on tasks, trouble planning ahead, trouble remembering the right word when talking, trouble understanding others, and headaches.

Background

Family Structure.   Married once. Living with wife, two sons (Sam, age 19; Stewart, age 10), one daughter (Jenifer, age 17).

Educational Background.   Attended 9 to 11 years of school; attended 3 or more years of trade school.

Military History.   In the National Guard from 1966 to 1974. Honorable discharge.

Employment History.   From 1962 to 1986, he was employed as a steamship clerk on the wharfs. A steamship clerk loads and discharges water or land vehicles which are transporting goods, and segregates cargo to be sure that it is going to the correct location. The job does not involve manual labor.

In 1984, Mr. Benson's gross pay was $56,540; in 1985, it was $44,330; in 1986, it was $24,105 for the first two quarters (he was injured in the second quarter). He did not collect a salary from August 11, 1986 through September 12, 1988 (gross pay was zero).

Psychiatric Hospitalization.   None reported or found in the available medical records before the incident. Was hospitalized six months after the exposure for an emotional breakdown after his house burnt down. Reports that his psychological symptoms were all present before this happened.

Outpatient Psychological Treatment.   None reported or found in the available medical records.

Medical History.   Non-contributory.

Hospitalization. Review of previous admissions were non-contributory. September 14, 1984. Discharge summary: atypical chest pain, probably musculoskeletal. No evidence of cardiac disease, February 21, 1983. Discharge summary: treatment of left hand for ammunition blow-up wound. June 17, 1983. Minor procedure to clean-up prior injury.

Alcohol Use. Mr. Benson reported infrequent use of alcohol, none at the present time.

Other Occupational or Domestic Neurotoxic Chemical Exposure. None found.

Family Neuropsychological-Related History. Father died of Parkinson's disease. Younger brother attempted suicide after a court ruling that his wife would get custody of the child after a divorce.

Personal References

1. K. Ganz, cousin, letter dated September 20, 1988. "John was a go-getter, never really tiring or getting bored as he has displayed since [the accident]. He has many episodes of depression . . . he cries . . . [he used to work] 50 to 70 hours a week . . . [now] he sleeps a lot or fidgets or gets angry or depressed. He now often likes to be alone—which is contrary to my knowledge of his past behavior . . . It is hard for John to swallow his present condition and to remain sane. The change happened almost immediately and not over a long period of time. To manifest and accept a new outlook on [his] performance/physical attributes is very hard for John."

2. T. Benson, letter undated. "Before the chemical accident my husband worked all the time. He was a workaholic. He worked sometimes 60 to 70 [hours] a week. He would shrimp in the Fall and do cabinet-making work whenever he could. He was always doing something in our house or in a friend's house. He was always very friendly, talked to everybody, joked and kidded around. He was always invited to go hunting, fishing, boating . . ."

General Observations

Initial impression. Stocky male, bearded, glasses, appeared his stated age. He was normally dressed. Speech was laconic.

General Demeanor. No abnormalities noted.

Posture and Gait. No abnormalities noted.

Involuntary Movements. No abnormalities noted.

Appearance. No abnormalities noted.

Speech. No abnormalities noted.

Thinking. Slowness.

Emotional State. Depressed, yet easily angered. He was brought to tears a few times during the interview (i.e., when describing that he wanted to harm himself or his children after his house burned down; and when describing the very frequent arguments between himself and his children).

Test-taking Behavior. Mr. Benson was cooperative and appeared to be trying to give his "best performance." He sat quietly, and his behavior was appropriate to the setting.

Previous Mental Function

Academic Records. Not available.

Emotional Functioning. Apparently normal.

Economic Functioning. Good.

Interpersonal Functioning. Apparently normal.

Pre-morbid IQ Estimation. Provisionally estimated at 105 (63rd percentile) based on current IQ.

Testing Standard. The 63rd percentile is provisionally used as a testing standard (estimate of pre-exposure global functioning). Scores at or below the 16th percentile are considered defective.

Neuropsychological Test Results and Interpretation

Wechsler Adult Intelligence Scale, Revised: WAIS-R

	Scaled Scores Age-Adjusted	Percentile Rank
Verbal Subscales		
Information	10	50
Digit Span	11	63
Vocabulary	10	50
Arithmetic	9	37
Comprehension	10	50
Similarities	12	75

Wechsler Adult Intelligence Scale, Revised: WAIS-R (Continued)

	Scaled Scores Age-Adjusted	Percentile Rank
Performance Subscales		
Picture Completion	15	95
Picture Arrangement	11	63
Block Design	15	95
Object Assembly	13	84
Digit Symbol	7	16*
Verbal IQ	99	47
Performance IQ	115	84
Full Scale IQ	105	63

*Deficit

Deficits were found in Digit Span (psychomotor speed, short-term memory).

Benton Visual Retention Test. This test assesses recent visual memory. Mr. Benson remembered eight designs, with two errors in reproduction; within normal limits.

The Embedded Figures Test. This test evaluates the ability to detect visual figure-ground relationships. Mr. Benson detected 37 of the 40 objects, within normal limits.

Grooved Pegboard Test. This test evaluates manual dexterity. Time for completion was 80 (17th percentile; *borderline defective*, right hand) and 71 seconds (60th percentile; left hand), within normal limits.

Trailmaking Test. This test evaluates visuomotor tracking and attention. Time for completing Part A was 33 seconds, the 32nd percentile. Time for completing Part B was 95 seconds, which is at the 28th percentile, borderline abnormal.

Controlled Oral Word Association Test. This test evaluates verbal fluency. Mr. Benson was *deficient* (5 to 8 percentile).

Wechsler Memory Scale: Logical Memory. Based upon an estimated premorbid verbal IQ of 105, it was expected that he would remember 23 elements upon immediate testing. Mr. Benson remembered 19 elements of the two stories upon immediate testing, which is *deficient* ($p < .03$). He remembered 15 elements upon delayed testing, *deficit in recent and delayed memory* ($p < .05$).

Paced Auditory Serial Addition Test. This test evaluates auditory information processing and tracking. Mr. Benson reproduced 22/60 correct responses, below the 1st percentile; *deficient in auditory information processing.*

Stroop Color and Word Test. This test evaluates mental flexibility. Mr. Benson scored at the 1st percentile for word reading (deficit in *psychomotor speed*), 11th percentile in color naming, and 4th percentile in Color/Word; *deficient in mental flexibility and psychomotor speed.*

Paired Associate Test. This test evaluates ability to learn. Mr. Benson performed within normal limits for recent memory, and *deficient for delayed memory* (at the 9th percentile).

Summary of Neuropsychologic Test Results

Deficit Functions. Deficits were found in numerous functions that are consistent with the diagnosis of neurotoxicity, including psychomotor speed, verbal fluency, recent and delayed memory auditory information processing, and mental flexibility.

Malingering Evaluation

Clinical Interview. No evidence for malingering was found in the course of the interview. Mr. Benson's account of his exposure and condition remained constant and did not fluctuate under questioning. His demeanor and affect were appropriate and credible. There was no evidence of exaggeration.

Test Performance. Test performance was credible. He performed at a very high level on some subtests.

Ungrouped Dot Counting Test. This test is used to assess malingering. It requires the patient to count the number of dots drawn on cards. The cards are presented in random order; if the patient is not malingering, it would take more time to count increasing number of dots. Responses were within normal limits.

Endorsement of Rare Symptoms. The Neurotoxicity Screening Survey presents seven symptoms that are rare. If a number of these symptoms are endorsed, the question of malingering is highlighted. Mr. Benson endorsed none.

Psychologic Functioning

Beck Depression Inventory. Mr. Benson showed mild-moderate depression.

Symptom Evaluation. Mr. Benson expressed symptoms in the following categories, which are indicative of neurotoxicity:

1. Personality changes
    a. Irritability
    b. Social withdrawal
    c. Amotivation (disturbance of executive function)
2. Mental changes
    a. Problems with memory for recent events
    b. Concentration difficulties
    c. Mental slowness
3. Sleep disturbance
4. Fatigue
5. Headache
6. Sexual dysfunction
7. Numbness in the hands or feet (depends upon the substance)
8. Recognition that there has been a loss of mental function

Neurophysiological Testing

Nerve conduction velocity of the median motor, median sensory and sural nerves on both sides was performed. The results are presented in Appendix I. Nerve conduction velocity was absent in both sural nerves. This is abnormal, and consistent with pesticide neurotoxicity.

Conclusions

Diagnosis. Brain damage (organic brain dysfunction), affecting emotional, interpersonal, and cognitive function.

Cause. Within reasonable scientific certainty, Thimet neurotoxicity caused, or was a significant contributing factor to, this disorder.

Prognosis. Guarded. Condition probably permanent.

APPENDIX
NERVE CONDUCTION VELOCITY

Name	John Benson					
Age	44					
Side	Left		Side	Right		
Temp.	Arm	28.83	Temp.	Arm		30.30
Temp.	Leg	28.25	Temp.	Leg		28.10

Name	John Benson				
Age	44				

Velocity Meters/sec—Right			Velocity Meters/sec—Left		
Median	Motor	54.49	Median	Motor	51.70
Median	Sensory	40.00	Median	Sensory	38.57
Sural		Abnormal	Sural		Abnormal

Amplitude (Motor in millivolts, sensory in microvolts)					
Median	Motor	21.20	Median	Motor	22.28
Median	Sensory	45.65	Median	Sensory	39.13
Sural		0.0	Sural		0.0

FORENSIC NEUROTOXICOLOGIC REPORT
OF
JOHN STRONG

John Strong was a 38 year old male evaluated on June 6, 1988 for nervous system and neuropsychological effects of exposure to pesticides.

Exposure.   On May 15, 1984, the patient was exposed to pesticides identified as Whitmire PT 250 and Dursban 2E.

Whitmire PT 250, according to the Material Safety Data Sheet, December 3, 1986, contains 99% solvents and propellents (methylene chloride, 1,1,1—trichloroethane) and 1% baygon (o-isopropoxyphenyl methylcarbamate).

Dursban 2E, according to the specimen label and the Material Safety Data Sheet, effective date October 16, 1985, contains 59.4% aromatic petroleum derivative solvent (xylene and other substances), 16.5% inert ingredients, and 24.1% chlorpyrifos (a trichloro-2-pyridyl phosphorothioate).

Initial impression.   No abnormalities noted. Mr. Strong appeared quiet and earnest.

Symptoms.   On the symptoms questionnaire, Mr. Strong endorsed many symptoms related to the nervous system, including problems with: memory, concentration, short attention span, easy distraction, excessive sleep, wakefulness, reduced sexual interest, fatigue, anxiety, depression, irritable, and loss of temper over trivial matters.

Background

Mr. Strong lives with his wife and child. He likes to work and be physically active, but is often fatigued now.

Educational Background.   Some college or technical school.

Employment History.   Mostly self-employed construction contractor.

Psychiatric Hospitalization.   None reported or found in the available medical records.

Outpatient Psychological Treatment.   None reported or found in the available medical records.

Hospitalization.   None reported or found in the available medical records.

Medical Records.   Pesticide poisoning.

Alcohol Use.   Moderate to heavy for a few years in the past; now some drinks a few times a year.

Other Occupational or Domestic Neurotoxic Chemical Exposure.   No significant exposures found. Some contract painting.

General Observations

General Demeanor.   No abnormalities noted.

Posture and Gait.   No abnormalities noted.

Involuntary Movements.   No abnormalities noted.

Appearance.   No abnormalities noted.

Speech.   No abnormalities noted.

Thinking.   Rate of thought production slow. Overly detailed descriptions.

Emotional State.   Somewhat depressed or else movements were slow due to sensory-motor dysfunction. Affect range restricted.

Previous Mental Function

Academic Records.   SAT: Verbal 459 (35th percentile), Math 508 (50th percentile) (5/68). Average 43rd percentile.

Pre-morbid IQ Estimation.   Estimated at 115, based on current best performance.

Neuropsychological Testing

Test-taking Behavior. Mr. Strong was cooperative and appeared to give an effort indicative of "best performance." He sat quietly, and his behavior was appropriate to the setting.

Test Results and Interpretation

Wechsler Adult Intelligence Scale, Revised: WAIS-R

	Scaled Scores Age-Adjusted	Percentile Rank
Verbal Subscales		
Information	14	91
Digit Span	8	25*
Vocabulary	12	75
Arithmetic	7	16*
Comprehension	13	84
Similarities	13	84
Performance Subscales		
Picture Completion	8	25*
Picture Arrangement	11	63
Block Design	10	50
Object Assembly	13	84
Digit Symbol	7	16*
Verbal IQ	107	
Performance IQ	93	
Full Scale IQ	100	

*Deficit

Current Mental Function

Mr. Strong's IQ was in the average range. Standard score of 13 used for comparison purposes (current best performance method) (84th percentile).

Deficits were found on Digit Span, Arithmetic, Picture completion, Object Assembly, and Digit Symbol Tests (*short-term memory, arithmetic, remote visual memory or visual perception, visuospatial organization, and psychomotor speed*).

Benton Visual Retention Test. This test assesses recent visual memory. Based upon a superior pre-morbid verbal IQ, 8 of 10 designs were expected to be correct, with 3 errors in reproduction. Mr. Strong remembered 8 designs, with 4 errors in reproduction; this was within normal limits.

The Embedded Figures Test. This test evaluates the ability to detect visual figure-ground relationships. Mr. Strong detected 36 of the 40 objects, 24th percentile, *deficit.*

Grooved Pegboard Test. This test evaluates manual dexterity. Time for completion was 65 and 81 seconds, 44th and 26th percentile.

Trailmaking Test. This test evaluates visuomotor tracking and attention. Time for completing Part A was 50 seconds, which is below the 1st percentile. Time for completing Part B was 89 seconds, which is below the 3rd percentile, *deficit in visuo-motor tracking, attention, and mental flexibility.*

Controlled Oral Word Association Test. This test evaluates verbal fluency. Mr. Strong scored in the severe deficit range (raw score 12), deficit in *verbal fluency.*

Wechsler Memory Scale: Logical Memory. Based upon an estimated premorbid verbal IQ of 110, it was expected that the subject would remember 25 elements upon immediate testing. Mr. Strong remembered 13 elements of the two stories upon immediate testing, which is *deficient* ($p < .0005$). He remembered 5 elements upon delayed testing, deficit in *recent and delayed memory.*

Paced Auditory Serial Addition Test. This test evaluates auditory information processing and tracking. Mr. Strong reproduced 19/60 correct responses, below the 1st percentile, deficit in *auditory information processing and tracking.*

Stroop Color and Word Test. This test evaluates mental flexibility. Mr. Strong scored at the 8th percentile for word reading (deficit in *psychomotor speed*), 5th percentile in color naming (deficit in *psychomotor speed*), and 1st percentile in Color/Word (deficit in *mental flexibility*).

Paired Associates Test. This test evaluates immediate and delayed memory. Mr. Strong scored at the 17th percentile, *deficit.*

Summary of Neuropsychologic Test Results: Numerous deficits consistent with pesticide and solvent neurotoxicity.

Malingering Evaluation

Clinical Interview. No evidence for malingering was found in the course of the interview. Mr. Strong's account of his exposure and condition remained constant and did not fluctuate under questioning. His demeanor and affect were appropriate and credible.

Test Performance.   Test performance was credible. He performed at a high level on many of the subtests.

Ungrouped Dot Counting.   This test is used to assess malingering. It requires the patient to count the number of dots drawn on cards. The cards are presented in random order; if the patient is not malingering, it would take more time to count an increasing number of dots. Responses were within normal limits.

Endorsement of Rare Symptoms.   The Neurotoxicity Screening Survey presents 7 symptoms that are rare. If a number of these symptoms are endorsed, the question of malingering is highlighted. Mr. Strong endorsed none of these.

Psychologic Function

Beck Depression Inventory.   Mr. Strong showed mild-moderate depression.

Profile of Mood Scale.

Mood	Percentile, Compared with Psychotherapy Outpatients
Tension	70
Depression	35
Anger	30
Vigilance	12
Fatigue	98
Confusion	86

Neurophysiological Testing

Nerve conduction velocity (NCV) tests of the median motor, median sensory and sural nerves on both sides were performed. The results are presented in Appendix I. NCV was slow and amplitudes low in both sural nerves.

Conclusions

Diagnosis.   Brain damage and nervous system dysfunction affecting cognitive, emotional and autonomic function.

Cause.   Within reasonable scientific certainty, neurotoxicity from pesticides caused or was a significant contributing factor to this disorder.

Prognosis.   Guarded. Condition probably permanent.

APPENDIX
NERVE CONDUCTION VELOCITY

Name	John Strong				
Age	38				

Side	Left		Side	Right	
Temp.	Arm	32.08	Temp.	Arm	32.65
Temp.	Leg	29.90	Temp.	Leg	28.20

	Velocity Meters/sec			Velocity Meters/sec	
Median	Motor	61.56	Median	Motor	61.33
Median	Sensory	53.43	Median	Sensory	49.72
Sural		38.87	Sural		35.00

	Amplitude (Motor in millivolts, sensory in microvolts)				
Median	Motor	11.96	Median	Motor	22.83
Median	Sensory	73.91	Median	Sensory	54.35
Sural		9.57	Sural		6.52

FORENSIC NEUROTOXICOLOGIC REPORT
OF
BILLY THOMPSON

Billy Thompson was a 41 year old male who was evaluated on February 19, 1985 and November 16, 1987 for residual nervous system and neuropsychological effects of exposure to PCBs, transformer liquid and related contaminants.

Exposure.   Mr. Thompson was exposed to transformer fluid containing PCBs from approximately 1970 to 1983. Before that time he had salvaged lead batteries from approximately 1967 to 1968. He had frequent dermal and respiratory contact with electrical transformer fluid and smoke from burning transformers.

Billy had been employed full time since 1970 at a metal salvage company, which currently is subject to federal litigation to enforce cleanup. The company had contracted with the state power company to retrofit the electrical transformers. The copper of the coils inside the transformers was valuable and was salvaged from the transformers. The copper was to be replaced with cheaper aluminum. Most of the transformers were 20 to 25 years old.

The transformers varied in size up to 1,000 gallons. The tops of the transformers were opened and the fluids were spilled on the ground. Transformer oil was wide spread on the property, equipment, hand tools, clothes, and exposed skin surfaces. It was estimated that 350,000 gallons of transformer fluid was dumped at that site.

The transformer coils were burned to remove the insulation. The smoke was described as gagging, wrenching, nauseating, caustic, searing, and it burned the eyes. Severe exposure to smoke occurred 2 to 3 times every month.

Initial Impression. Billy's demeanor was friendly, open, and helpful. He was overweight, quiet, and calm. He seemed to have visuo-spatial difficulties when walking, and when he arranged boxes in the trunk of a car. Physical production of speech was normal. No unusual physical mannerisms were noted.

Interview (November 16, 1987). Billy said that he felt needles sticking in his hands, particularly the left hand. He reported that certain people had control over his hands, but when he tried to give details about the sensation, he had difficulty with the description. He had been living in his truck since I had last examined him. When asleep, he saw what he called "movies." In one of these "movies" he went to Halstead Air Force Base, and a lady told him to wear a suit (I had been looking at his unkempt, disheveled clothing). She said that his name had been selected from "the service list, child support thing . . . I don't know who did it, I wasn't supposed to be put out of my house in the first place."

When questioned about this "dream," fantasy or hallucination, he said that "In my opinion, it's a movie; most people say it is a dream. If you don't have knowledge, you say it's a dream. Now you can tell a dream, but a movie is different altogether." The story continued with a loose plot, involving the Navy, Marines, Air Force, and President Reagan.

When asked about a typical day, he had some problems organizing his thoughts, and needed many questions to elicit an orderly flow of information. He did not work, but he did collect aluminum cans for redemption. He did not talk much to anyone, although he did see some friends. He seemed to have the rudiments of friendship without the substance or content. He basically stayed in his truck, where he lived, near his uncle. He had no money to ride buses, so he traveled only when someone offered him a ride. His only income was from "beer picking." He has not tried to get any assistance—thoughts (not voices) tell him not to travel too far.

When asked if he heard voices, Billy replied that he saw visual pictures, not hallucinations, such as Henry Kissinger telling him things, then Billy continued with a long, rambling story.

Symptoms. On the symptom questionnaire, Billy had endorsed many symptoms related to the nervous system, including problems with memory, concentration, attention, thinking quickly and clearly, fatigue, and numbness and tingling in the arms and feet.

Background

Billy was divorced, had two children, and lived alone. His wife had left him because of his violent and erratic behavior. His wife had testified that they had slept apart for a number of years because Billy slept restlessly, and also had a problem with lack of erections.

Educational Background. Billy had had some high school education and had gotten a GED at age 16 or 17.

Employment History. He had worked as a truck driver for many years.

Psychiatric Hospitalization. None reported or found in the available medical records.

Outpatient Psychological Treatment. Billy had been briefly treated for alcohol abuse following a driving while intoxicated (DWI) incident. This occurred when his wife had left him. There was possibly some psychotic behavior of his brother and/or father.

Hospitalization. None reported.

Alcohol Use. Billy reported infrequent use of alcohol, prior to the DWI incident. At the time of his examination he said that he did not drink.

General Observations

General Demeanor. Friendly, helpful, simple.

Posture and Gait. Some problems with walking (visuo-spatial).

Involuntary Movements. None were noticeable.

Appearance. Billy Thompson was dressed in a mildly disheveled manner.

Speech. Some misuse and confusion of words.

Thinking. Mental confusion, tangential associations, lack of clarity and coherence.

Emotional State. Billy appeared to be in mental distress. He was aware of his problems but did not see any solutions to his difficulties.

Previous Mental Function

Academic Records.   Not available.

Personal References.

1. Helen Janko. Oral statement, November 16, 1987. This is the wife of the subject's cousin, and has known Billy more than 20 years. ". . . I used to see him pretty often, but haven't seen him for the last 3 years. There was a big change in Billy that started about 4 to 5 years ago. It seems like something was happening to his mind. He started to see and hear things that no one else knew about. Before becoming sick, as far as I know, he had friends. He was an outgoing guy, he was always there if we needed something. He was very friendly, and honest, as far as I know. He seemed to be OK with his children. He was a guy who was really concerned about his family. About 4 to 5 years ago, he began to talk a lot that didn't make sense. He would go on all day long. I heard that now he lives in his truck. I've even passed by there but I've never seen him."

2. Tom Water of Tom Water Enterprise. Oral statement November 16, 1987. ". . . I've known Billy for 10 years. I saw him a month ago. Billy used to be a driver for the Reclamation Company, that's how I knew him. Billy has undergone big changes. I think he went wacko. He said that the insurance man put the devil in him, and that someone is controlling him. Before he was sick, he was just a normal person. He was like everyone else. He was a good truck driver. When he came by, he would stop and say hello. His wife left him after the devil got in him. Billy is not a drinker. He really believes that there is something inside him. Once he said that they got him last night—sometimes he says it hurts so bad he can't stand it. There's been a considerable change in Billy in the past 8 years. Before that time there was no indication of his being sick. As far as I know, he had to be reliable to be working on the same job for years. Now he is not capable of being on the road. There's a big change in the man."

3. Jed Handy, Handy Towing and Trucking Company. February 6, 1985, written statement "Mr. Billy Thompson can no longer work or perform his truck driving abilities like he has done in the past."

4. Ben Washing, currently at Marine Run Limited. Oral statement, November 16, 1987. "Billy was an owner-operator who worked for his company [after he stopped working for the Reclamation Company—see W. Dest] I haven't seen Billy for a number of years. He was a good worker when he was able to work. Frequently was spaced out. He was not a drinker, smoker, or abuser of substances."

5. W. Dest. Oral statement, November 16, 1987. "I've known Billy around 7 or 8 years. We met on the same job. Billy was working for Transport, Inc.,

after working for the Reclamation Company. We worked together from 1980 to 1982. I've seen him on and off since then. During the time we worked together, he was OK. He was very dependable. He got along well with all the other guys. I don't see Billy much now. He ain't the same since I once knew him. Billy was a worker. When I see his truck with bushes growing around it, I know that's not Billy.''

6. F. Fellow. Oral statement, December 10, 1987. "Billy Thompson is 10% the man he was. He was not above normal intelligence, but his memory was excellent—he could remember names, places, things. I talked to Billy 3 months ago; he is degenerating. He is hard to converse with.''

7. N. Green. Written statement, February 26, 1985. This was Billy's friend. "Billy Thompson can't function in his work like he used to.''

Using Barona and Chastain's 1986 formula for predicting premorbid IQ, it was calculated that Billy Thompson's verbal IQ was 91 (27th percentile)—Average, Performance IQ at 84 (15th percentile)—Low Average, and Full Scale IQ was at 90 (25th percentile)—Average.

Estimation. The achievement of a GED, the demographic formula, Billy Thompson's references and probable work performance indicate a prior mental function of Average to Low Average.

Examination

Test-taking Behavior. Mr. Thompson was cooperative and appeared to give an effort indicative of "best performance." He sat quietly, and his behavior was appropriate to the setting.

Test Results and Interpretation

Wechsler Adult Intelligence Scale, Revised: WAIS-R

	Testing August 16, 1987 Scaled Scores Percentile		Testing August 19, 1985 Scaled Scores Percentile	
	Age-Adjusted	Rank	Age-Adjusted	Rank
Verbal Subscales				
Information	6	9	6	9
Digit Span	10	50	7	16
Vocabulary	5	5	4	2
Arithmetic	6	5	6	9
Comprehension	7	16	7	16
Similarities	4	2	5	5

Wechsler Adult Intelligence Scale, Revised: WAIS-R (Continued)

	Testing August 16, 1987 Scaled Scores Percentile		Testing August 19, 1985 Scaled Scores Percentile	
	Age-Adjusted	Rank	Age-Adjusted	Rank
Performance Subscales				
Picture Completion	7	16	6	9
Picture Arrangement	5	5	8	25
Block Design	6	5	5	5
Object Assembly	6	9	5	5
Digit Symbol	5	5	5	5
Verbal IQ	78	7 (Borderline)	78	7
Performance IQ	74	4 (Borderline)	74	4
Full Scale IQ	75	5 (Borderline)	75	5

Current Mental Function

Billy Thompson's IQ was in the borderline range. There was an overall drop in IQ of 15 points from estimated pre-morbid status. However, his IQ had not changed since the first test.

In the Verbal section of the WAIS-R, a deficit was found in the Digit Span Subtest, indicating a deficit in *short-term memory*. The subject could only reliably remember two digits in the backwards direction. This was the same performance as found previously.

Benton Visual Retention Test.   This test assesses recent visual memory. Based upon a low average pre-morbid verbal IQ, 7 of 10 designs were expected to be correct, with 4 errors in reproduction. The subject remembered 6 designs, with 10 errors in reproduction, indicating *impairment of visual memory*. In the previous test, he had remembered 1 design with 15 errors.

The Embedded Figures Test.   This test evaluates the ability to detect visual figure-ground relationships. Billy Thompson detected 19 of the 40 objects, below the 1st percentile, *deficit in visual figure-ground perception*. Previously he had seen 24 objects.

Grooved Pegboard Test.   This test evaluates manual dexterity. The time for completion was 84 seconds for the dominant hand, which is approximately at the 6th percentile, and 94 seconds for the nondominant hand, which is approximately at the 6th percentile. This shows a *deficit in manual dexterity*. Previously his times were 80 and 108 seconds.

Trailmaking Test. This test evaluates visuomotor tracking and attention. Time for completing Part A was 126 seconds, which is below the 1st percentile. Time for completing Part B was 378 seconds, which is below the 1st percentile. This denotes a *deficit in visuo-motor tracking, attention, and mental flexibility*. Previously his time on Part A had been 96. He could not complete Part B because of confusion.

Controlled Oral Word Association Test. This test evaluates verbal fluency. Billy Thompson's performance was measured below the 1st percentile, showing a *deficit in verbal fluency*. This was the same result as had appeared when he had been previously tested.

Wechsler Memory Scale: Logical Memory. This test was administered on February 19, 1985. Based upon a premorbid Verbal IQ in the average range (90), it was expected that he would remember 18 elements upon immediate testing, and 8 elements upon delayed testing. The subject remembered only 9 elements of the 2 stories upon immediate testing, which indicates a deficiency ($p <$ .0005) in *recent verbal memory* for logically related elements. The subject remembered 6 elements upon delayed testing, which was expected when only 9 elements are initially remembered.

Test Results

Deficits. The same deficits found previously were found upon reexamination: Overall IQ, memory, visual perception, manual dexterity, and verbal fluency.

Malingering Evaluation

Clinical Interview. No evidence for malingering was found in the course of the interview.

Test Performance. Test performance was credible. Note that the exact same overall IQ was found for the two testing sessions, more than 2 years apart.

Ungrouped Dot Counting. This test is used to assess malingering. It requires the patient to count the number of dots drawn on cards. The cards are presented in a random order; if the patient is not malingering, it takes more time to count an increasing number of dots. The subject's responses were within normal limits. The same results had been found previously.

Memorization of "15" Items.   This test is used to assess malingering. Malingering was not found. The test was administered on February 19, 1985.

Psychologic Function

Billy was found to be severely mentally disturbed, with many life functioning difficulties.

Neurophysiological Testing

Nerve conduction velocity of the median motor, median sensory and sural nerves on both sides was performed. The results are presented in Appendix 1. Nerve conduction velocity slowing was found in the left sural nerve (32 m/s), and reduced amplitude of the right sural nerve. Previous testing found reduced amplitude of the right median sensory and sural nerves.

Conclusion

Within reasonable scientific certainty, Billy Thompson was suffering from neuropsychological dysfunction associated with exposure to PCB transformer fluid and related contaminants. Although there was exposure to lead prior to exposure to PCBs, Billy had apparently been functioning adequately before exposure to PCB and related contaminants. Co-workers who were examined and who had not been exposed to lead were also found to have the symptoms and signs of neurotoxicity related to PCB exposure.

APPENDIX
NERVE CONDUCTION VELOCITY

Name	Billy Thompson		November 16, 1987		
Age	41				
Side	Left		Side	Right	
Temp.	Arm	32.88	Temp.	Arm	31.25
Temp.	Leg	28.10	Temp.	Leg	27.85
	Velocity Meters/Sec			Velocity Meters/Sec	
Median	Motor		Median	Motor	Not Measured
Median	Sensory	54.12	Median	Sensory	45.43
Sural		32.35	Sural		41.82

Name	Billy Thompson		November 16, 1987		
Age	41				
Amplitude (Motor in Millevolts, Sensory in Microvolts)					
Median	Sensory	47.83	Median	Sensory	47.83
Sural		41.30	Sural		8.70

Name	Billy Thompson		February 19, 1985		
Age	38				
Side	Left		Side	Right	
Temp.	Arm	32.65	Temp.	Arm	32.90
Temp.	Leg	30.10	Temp.	Leg	29.85
Velocity Meters/Sec			Velocity Meters/Sec		
Median	Motor	62.67	Median	Motor	61.40
Median	Sensory	50.00	Median	Sensory	47.03
Sural		44.91	Sural		45.56
Amplitude (Motor in Millevolts, Sensory in Microvolts)					
Median	Motor	5.00	Median	Motor	5.65
Median	Sensory	17.39	Median	Sensory	13.04
Sural		11.96	Sural		7.61

NEUROTOXICITY EVALUATION OF GREGORY DEPARK

Gregory Depark was a 59 year old man who worked as a truck repairman and spray painter for the United States government for 15 years, until November 1983. At that job, paint fumes often were inhaled by spray painters and bystanders. The fumes contain mixed solvents, dyes and other additives, such as lead. Mr. Depark, who used only a small white mask for protection, was exposed to paint spray on a daily basis.

Since 1972, the facility at which Mr. Depark worked had used a lead-based enamel paint on its trucks. Beginning around 1980 or 1981, Mr. Depark suffered from severe headaches, dizziness, and vomiting. In October 1983, the subject suffered a heart attack, and was hospitalized for 2 or 3 weeks. He then underwent lead chelation, because he had shown elevated lead levels. The chelation treatment apparently alleviated the headaches and vomiting, but the subject still suffered from dizzy spells.

Examination

I examined Mr. Depark in December 1984 and January 1985, and treated him for about a year. Mr. Depark, who was prone to confusion and disorientation, was initially driven by his brother. The subject was very well-mannered and gentlemanly. He did not know the date but knew the day, month, and year. His speech was halting. He often had difficulty finding words to express himself.

When asked to write a sentence, he wrote "I wish I could find something useful to do," expressing his wish to once again be a productive member of society.

Mr. Depark said that his main problems were that he "could not concentrate," that he was anxious and depressed, and that he didn't "have the volition to do anything." He reported having these symptoms for the past four years. He said that he doesn't "seem to have a goal. Sometimes I'm interested in something, but 15 minutes later I'm exhausted." He has trouble organizing and understanding tools that he had been able to use for many years before his perceived change in mental ability. He was troubled by headaches, nausea and he vomited bile.

Mr. Depark was noticeably uncoordinated in gate and balance. He was not confident about the location of his feet. Mr. Depark reported that his left leg "collapsed out from under" him. This occured every few days, perhaps three or four times a day.

Mr. Depark had serious problems with memory, affecting all aspects of his life. He forgot where he was going, and why he was going there. He misnamed the month of the examination and his time sense was also distorted. Guessing the time, shortly after he arrived for the examination, was wrong by two hours. He also had trouble concentrating, and reported being easily distracted and finding it hard to think clearly. He was troubled by his difficulty in finding words and understanding speech and writing.

Mr. Depark had panic attacks, which seemed to have subsided somewhat after chelation therapy. He also had weakness, tremors and shakiness in his arms and legs.

Sexual dysfunction troubled him. Erections were difficult to achieve. Sexual relations occured about once every two weeks. These problems began about two years before his treatment. Although heart medication was begun one year before treatment, no change in this problem was noted at the time. Sexual function had been steadily decreasing.

Educational and Vocational Background

Mr. Depark attended one and a half years of high school, but he could not continue because he had to work to support himself. Later he attended County Community College for one year, where he studied anatomy, physiology, microbiology, trigonometry and physics; but he could not afford to continue his studies. He maintained a B grade-point average.

Mr. Depark holds a number of U.S. patents. In 1951, he was awarded a patent for "apparatus and methods for molding concrete vaults and the like." In 1953, he was awarded a patent for an "hydraulic vibratory cylinder." In 1965, he was awarded a patent for a "fluid operated motor vehicle lifting jack." The schematic drawings for these patents were very complicated. Mr. Depark reported that he cannot understand these drawings anymore. Other symptoms of loss of function included his reported inability to fix his own car; he also reported difficulty with simple tools such as screwdrivers.

Mr. Depark used to like to read; at the time of his examination he said that he did not know what many words meant, and that he had trouble keeping his eyes on the lines. High levels of lead were found in his blood in 1984. These levels were reduced following chelation for lead.

Test Results

Wechsler Adult Intelligence Scale, Revised: WAIS-R

	IQ	
Verbal Scale	96	Average
Non-verbal Scale (Performance)	93	Average
Full Scale Intelligence	94	Average
	Subscale scores (age-adjusted)	Percentile rank
Verbal Subscales		
Information	13	84
Digit Span	7	16
Vocabulary	10	50
Arithmetic	10	50
Comprehension	10	50
Similarities	9	37
Nonverbal Subscales		
Picture Completion	9	37
Block Design	8	25
Object Assembly	11	63
Digit Symbol	8	25

Interpretation of Neuropsychologic Findings

Wechsler Intelligence Scale, Revised.   Deficits were seen in Digit Span (immediate memory); Digit Symbol (psychomotor speed) and Block Design (visuospatial function).

The Embedded Figures Test.   This test assesses the patient's ability to discriminate figure from ground in a visually distracting field. The test consists of four cards, presented one at a time, on which are overlapping line drawings of ten common objects. The patient is asked to name the objects and is given 60 seconds to do so. Visual perception deficit was found.

Memorization of 15 Items.   This test is used to assess the validity of a memory complaint. Only the most severely brain damaged or retarded person would fail this test, unless there was a conscious or unconscious attempt to fail. A deficit was found.

The Ungrouped Dot Counting Test.   This test is used to assess malingering. The patient has to count the number of dots presented on cards. The cards are presented in a random order; if the patient is not malingering, it would take more time to count increasing number of dots. Malingering was not found.

The Benton Visual Retention Test.   This test assesses the ability to remember and reproduce geometric shapes. Administration B; Form C Number Correct 4; Errors 8. Mr. Depark was deficient in visual perception and memory.

The Grooved Pegboard Test.   This test assesses manual dexterity by timing the patient as he or she manipulates pegs into grooved slots. No abnormalities were noted. Right hand dominant. Right hand: 73 seconds. Left hand: 86 seconds.

Controlled Word Association Test.   This test assesses the ability to access words. Marked verbal fluency deficit was found.

Wechsler Memory Scale.   This test assesses recent and delayed memory. Mr. Depark was found to have short-term memory deficit.

Immediate Recall:	Predicted for verbal IQ 95:	19
	Observed	12
	Residual	7
	Probability of Residual	.005
	Memory Deficit	
Delayed Recall:	Predicted for immediate recall of 12:	11
	Observed	9
	Residual	2
	Probability of Residual	.1

Summary of Neuropsychologic Findings

Mr. Depark showed deficits which suggest diffuse brain dysfunction.

Neurophysiologic Findings

The nerve conduction velocity (NCV) of the median motor, median sensory and sural (sensory) nerves were assessed. Median motor NCV was measured from elbow to wrist; median sensory NCV was measured from wrist to index finger; and sural NCV was measured from the calf to heel. The results were as follows:

Nerve	Side	Velocity (Meters/Second)	Temperature (Centigrade)
Median motor	Left	49	30
Median sensory	Left	35	30
Sural	Left	Absent	
Median motor	Right	49	29
Median sensory	Right	30	29
Sural	Right	Absent	

The sural nerve response was absent, which indicates peripheral nerve dysfunction characteristic of neurotoxic chemical exposure.

Summary

Neural dysfunction indicative of neurotoxicity was found. Deterioration in personality, perception, sexual function, memory, and concentration were severe. The most probable cause of this dysfunction was toxic chemical exposure at the worksite including exposure to spray paint consisting of solvents and lead pigment.

Prognosis

The deterioration over the past few years is likely to continue. Because brain cells do not regenerate, improvement in mental function is not usually expected. However, to maximize present capacity and to promote a healthful lifestyle, I recommended treatment including neuropsychologic counseling and rehabilitation, physical therapy, and avoidance of toxic chemicals in food and the environment.

NEUROTOXICOLOGIC AND NEUROPSYCHOLOGIC EVALUATION
OF
KENNETH DEFOREST

Kenneth Deforest was a 41 year old male evaluated on April 4, 1987 for residual nervous system effects from exposure to hydrogen sulfide.

Exposure

On February 8, 1987, at approximately 9 A.M., five fishermen set out to fish at a sulphur mining rig in the Gulf of Mexico. The boat was 32 feet by 12 feet. Local fishermen often fish near the rigs, as the fish seem to be attracted to the rigs, perhaps because it is a source of sea life which cling to the undersea rig apparatus.

At approximately 9:20 A.M., the men arrived at the rig and tied their boat to a cable associated with the rig. The smell of ''sulphur'' was present. The fishermen saw and heard 2 1/2 feet diameter gas bubbles coming to the surface. Soon, one fisherman passed out. Within about 10 seconds, the remaining fishermen passed out. At 10:10 A.M., a boater who was passing by radioed the Coast Guard for help. At 10:30 A.M., the Coast Guard found that the boat had run aground, and they assisted in refloatation of the boat. The total time that the men had been unconscious was about 20 to 50 minutes. They were taken to a local hospital for treatment, where they were diagnosed to have been suffering from toxic fume inhalation.

The rig to which the fishermen had tied their boat used the Frasch process to mine sulphur. This process is used when sulphur is mined far below the surface. A hole is drilled using petroleum drilling apparatus, and three concentric pipes are lowered into the cavity. Through one pipe, steam is forced down; through another, water is forced down, and through a third, the liquid sulphur/water mix is brought to the surface.

Whenever sulphur is mined, there is always the possibility that hydrogen sulfide will be present. Hydrogen sulfide may bubble up if there is gap in the well piping or if the removal of the sulpher creates a void or space where hydrogen sulfide gas can migrate through porous media (the rock types). Once the sulphur reaches the sea floor, it will rise to the surface because it is lighter than water.

Initial Impression.   Mr. Deforest appeared to be serious. He was dressed casually and neatly for the examination. He was cooperative and seemed to answer the questions to the best of his ability.

Symptoms. Mr. Deforest reported suffering from anxiety, depression, irritability, confusion, headaches, and fatigue; he also reported problems with memory, concentration, and sleep.

Medical History. Previous medical history was noncontributory.

Previous Mental Function. Mr. Deforest maintained approximately a B average in college, suggesting an above average mental ability before the exposure. A Full Scale IQ of 107 (68th percentile) was calculated using Barona and Chastain's 1986 demographic formula for estimating premorbid IQ. Test data interpretation was based on an estimated Full Scale IQ of 107 and a scaled score of 11.

Test-Taking Behavior. Mr. Deforest was cooperative and appeared to be performing at his best. The test administrator did not have the impression that he was malingering.

Test Results and Interpretation

Wechsler Adult Intelligence Scale, Revised: WAIS-R

	Scaled Scores	Percentile Rank Age-Adjusted	
Verbal Subscales			
Information	8	25	
Digit Span	10	50	
Vocabulary	8	25	
Arithmetic	9	37	
Comprehension	10	50	
Similarities	8	25	
Nonverbal Subscales			
Picture Completion	9	37	
Picture Arrangement	8	25	
Block Design	9	37	
Object Assembly	13	84	
Digit Symbol	10	50	
Verbal IQ	91	27th	Average
Performance IQ	97	42nd	Average
Full Scale IQ	93	32nd	Average

Current Mental Function.   In the Verbal Section of the WAIS-R, a deficit was found in Digits Backward, indicating a deficit in *short-term memory*. Mr. Deforest could only reliably remember three digits in the backwards direction.

Benton Visual Retention Test.   This test assesses recent visual memory. Based upon Mr. Deforest's estimated premorbid IQ in the average range (107), 7 of 10 designs were expected to be correct, with 4 errors in reproduction. Mr. Deforest remembered 4 designs, with 9 errors in reproduction. The correct score suggests impairment and the error score strongly indicates impairment of *recent visual memory*.

Wechsler Memory Scale: Logical Memory.   Based upon Mr. Deforest's estimated premorbid verbal IQ (calculated using Barona et al.) in the average range (107), it was expected that he would remember 23 elements upon immediate testing, and 11 elements upon delayed testing. Mr. Deforest remembered only 12 elements of the two stories upon immediate testing, indicating a deficiency ($p < .0005$) in *recent verbal memory* for logically related elements. In addition, Mr. Deforest remembered only 6 elements upon delayed testing, indicating a deficit ($p < .019$) in *delayed verbal memory* for recently learned materials.

The Embedded Figures Test.   This test evaluates the ability to detect visual figure-ground relationships. Mr. Deforest detected 27 of the 40 objects, which is approximately at the 12th percentile, a deficit in *detecting figure-ground* relationships.

Grooved Pegboard Test.   This test evaluates manual dexterity. Time for completion was 72 seconds for the dominant hand, which is approximately at the 42nd percentile, and 76 seconds for the non-dominant hand, which is approximately at the 44th percentile, both within normal range.

Trailmaking Test.   This test evaluates visuomotor tracking and attention. Time for completing Part A was 43 seconds, which is approximately at the 7th percentile, a deficit in *visuomotor tracking and attention*. Time for completing Part B was 68 seconds, which is approximately at the 67th percentile, within normal range.

Paced Auditory Serial Addition Test.   This test evaluates *auditory information processing and tracking*. The results of this test indicated that Mr. Deforest was below the 1st percentile ($p < .003$), a deficit.

Controlled Oral Word Association Test. This test evaluates verbal fluency. Mr. Deforest's performance was measured at the 20th percentile, a possible deficit in *verbal fluency.*

Gordon Diagnostic System. This diagnostic device was used to assess vigilance, distractibility, and malingering.

Vigilance. Within normal range.

Distractibility. Within normal range.

Malingering. Not indicated.

Test Results

A possible decline in overall WAIS-R IQ was found.

Specific deficits were found in recent short-term memory, recent visual memory, recent and delayed auditory logical memory, visuomotor tracking, and auditory attention and information processing and tracking.

Malingering Tests

Clinical Interview. No evidence for malingering was found in the course of the interview.

Minnesota Multiphasic Personality Inventory (MMPI). This test was used to assess malingering and psychological state. Malingering was not indicated on this test.

Gordon Diagnostic System. Results presented previously in this report.

Conclusion

Within reasonable scientific certainty, Kenneth Deforest was suffering from neuropsychological dysfunction related to hydrogen sulfide exposure. Similar results were found in his companions on the boat.

It was recommended that Mr. Deforest receive psychotherapy on a weekly basis. The focus of the therapy was to be on having him confront his experience surrounding the accident, and on accepting and adjusting to his decline in neuropsychological abilities. It was also recommended that he have vocational rehabilitation because he may have difficulty with the cognitive and emotional demands of many occupations, and he should not work in an environment where he would be exposed to neurotoxic chemicals in the future.

APPENDIX
NEUROTOXICITY OF HYDROGEN SULFIDE

Hydrogen sulfide is an established inhibitor of cytochrome oxidase in vitro. Signs and symptoms of poisoning resemble cyanide poisoning. Hydrogen sulfide also forms a complex with methemoglobin known as sulfmethemoglobin, which is analogous to cyanmethemoglobin. Poisoning leads to histotoxic hypoxia. This term is somewhat misleading, because the toxic effect does not result from an inadequate supply of oxygen, but from an inability of cells to use oxygen (Smith, 1986).

Although the exact chemical details are still unknown, the undissociated form of hydrogen sulfide appears to block electron transfer in the cytochrome a-a3 complex, which is isolated in vitro as a single unit. As a consequence, oxygen metabolism is compromised, so that it cannot meet metabolic demands. At the level of the brain stem nuclei, this effect may result in central respiratory arrest and death (Smith, 1986).

Systemic poisoning at exposures of 500 to 2000 ppm primarily targets the nervous system. After a single exposure of 2000 ppm or more, unconsciousness occurs within a few seconds, without significant warning or pain, almost immediately followed by respiratory paralysis, and after that by a short period of tonic convulsions (Gosselin et al. 1984). The heart continues to beat for a few minutes. Death occurs unless the victim is removed from the contaminated area.

Lethal hydrogen sulfide poisoning exerts its effect directly on the nervous system. If the concentration of the gas is sufficiently high, the respiratory center of the brain ceases to function and breathing stops. At concentrations of 500 to 1000 ppm, the autonomic controls of respiration whose sensors are in the carotid body are stimulated, resulting in hypernea, followed by apnea, resulting from instigation of the normal autonomic reflex.

Survivors of acute toxic episodes sometimes show neurologic sequelae such as amnesia, intention tremor, neurasthenia, disturbance of equilibrium or more serious brain stem and cortical damage, but complete recovery is thought to usually occur (Gosselin et al. 1984). However, hypoxic tissue damage can occur, producing neurologic deficits like those occurring in survivors of other severe asphyxiant poisonings, for example with carbon monoxide and cyanide.

REFERENCES

Smith, R. P. 1986. Toxic responses of the blood. In Casarett and Doull's *Toxicology; The Basic Sciences of Poisons*, 3rd Ed. Eds. Curtis D. Klaassen, Mary O. Amdur, and John Doull. New York: Macmillan Publishing Company.

Gosselin, R. E., Smith, R. P., Hodge, H. C. 1984, *Clinical Toxicology of Commercial Products*, 5th Ed. Section III. Baltimore: Williams & Wilkins.

FORMALDEHYDE CASE REPORT 1
UREA FORMALDEHYDE FOAM INSULATION EXPOSURE OF
ELLEN WHITE

Ellen White was a 57 year old female evaluated on April 10, 1987 for residual nervous system effects from exposure to urea formaldehyde foam insulation (UFFI).

In 1979, Ms. White moved into an apartment which previously had been insulated with UFFI. She became fatigued, and often had a sore throat, dry nose, sores in her nose, and felt achy and tired.

In December 1981, the apartment roof began to leak. Water leaked down a closet wall. Maintenance workers cut a hole in the closet to let the warm air up to the roof to melt the ice. Unfortunately, this hole was also a conduit for UFFI fumes.

Ms. White fell on ice in January 1982, and had to stay home because she could not walk. At home she had flu-like symptoms and stayed in bed. She reported that her cats developed allergies. If a human is affected by pollutants in a home, it is likely that pets will also be affected.

When Ms. White returned to work, she was fatigued, and was sensitive to ammonia and cigarette fumes. She seemed to recover somewhat when away from the apartment for a few days.

Exposure Testing. An industrial hygienist reviewed the exposure situation; the following information is taken from his report. The only available readings for formaldehyde levels are from July 28, 1982 (exposure began in 1979). The readings ranged from 0.09 to 0.24 ppm. These levels are above the ASHRAE standard of 0.10 ppm. Because highest levels of formaldehyde occur within the first six months after UFFI insulation exposure, it was likely that formaldehyde levels were higher in 1979 than they were in 1982.

However, the highest exposure levels probably occurred in December 1981, when the apartment had water damage, and a portion of the external wall which contained UFFI was opened up by maintenance workers.

Water damage increases the hydrolysis in foam and therefore increases the emission of formaldehyde. Depending upon the extent of the wetting of the UFFI, and temperatures at the time, formaldehyde levels, and consequently, exposures, may have been at twice the level, or more, above what is considered normal for homes with UFFI.

Formaldehyde levels inside wall cavities are typically several ppm. The opening of the wall cavity in the White apartment would have caused a ''burst'' of 1 ppm or more in the adjacent room. It also would have resulted in continued elevated levels for as long as the hole was opened.

Previous Levels of Activity.   Ms. White said that before moving into the apartment, she customarily got up at 5 A.M., had coffee and then went to work. She had been very active in a folk dance group, and entertained twice a week. At the time of her examination she neither danced or entertained.

Symptoms.   Ms. White reported anxiety, depression, irritability, feelings of helplessness, mood changes, worry, loss of sexual interest, distractibility, trouble beginning tasks, trouble with planning, problems with memory, headaches, problems with sleep, tiredness, fatigue, trouble using tools, muscle weakness in arms, hands, legs, and feet, numbness and tingling in legs, loss of feeling in feet, reduction and change in sense of smell, reduction in sense of taste, moving in a jerky or uneven manner (drags right foot), and difficulty turning over in bed.

Psychosocial History.   Ms. White was divorced and had one child. At the time of the examination she lived alone in an environmentally restricted atmosphere, and rarely left her home.

Alcohol Use.   Ms. White reported that until 1982 she drank alcohol a few times a year; in 1982 she stopped drinking alcohol.

Medication.   Ms. White had taken anti-convulsant medication, primarily dilantin and phenobarbital, from the 1960s to 1985. She had a history of nocturnal spasms, which may have been sleep apnea. At the time of her examination she took phenobarbital (an anti-convulsant), ventilin and seldane (for respiratory problems). She was on minimum medication during the examination.

Employment History.   Between 1972 and 1982, Ms. White worked in various executive positions, primarily with non-profit or political groups. Her jobs required contact with the public, and a high level of organizational and communication skills. Occupational exposure to neurotoxic agents was not found.

Personal References.   Letter from an associate who had known Ms. White for 15 years. They worked together in a well-known a consumer oriented organization. "Ellen was creative, energetic and resourceful, and her know-how in public relations helped attract volunteers from various professions . . . What might have been viewed as insurmountable tasks by persons less able were accomplished by Ellen by means of excellent skills and insight, plus a great deal of hard work . . . (She had a zest for living; was an active member of the Church, joining the folkdance group and the choir). In contrast to the vital person I remember from the 1970s is the very different Ellen White, who in recent years, through circumstances well beyond her control has been forced into the existence of a recluse . . .''

Election results for State Citizen of the Year—1974, selected by editors of the state's seven leading newspapers. Ellen placed third. (A former governor of the state, placed first). The editor of *The Capitol Times* nominated Ms. White, saying ''. . . Ellen White, who is Executive Director of . . . in this state, speaks for one of the largest groups in the state, and it seems to me that her effectiveness goes beyond her constituency and deals really with her expertise and her study of the issues. She's a person who knows how to speak to power, and also, how to speak to the public which is at the root of power. And I nominate Ellen White not only on her own right, but as a representative of the growing number of citizen lobbyists who, I think, play an increasingly vital role in working for good government.''

Letter from the governor of the state appointing Ms. White to the Citizen Advisory Committee to the Regional States River Basins Program.

College Graduate Center Newsletter, June–July 1977. ''50th Management Development Program Class Elects First Woman President,'' Ms. White.

Letter from state governor, 1972. Personal letter of thanks for her work.

Lakeville Journal, April 27, 1972. ''One Citizen Can Make A Difference: How White Helped Save Wetlands.''

Kodak job evaluation. Ms. White was a Service Clerk Dispatcher. A critical, but generally favorable, report on her work performance. References are made to her illness.

Medical Reports.   Her treating physician reported that Ms. White had the following conditions: hyperreactive airway syndrome, depression, upper respiratory allergies and irritability, manifested by spasmodic coughing, episodic nosebleeds and nasal congestion. The patient's main disability remains emotional—reactive depression because of her illness and loss of self-esteem related to her loss of work and inability to engage in productive work.

Specialized testing found decreased olfactory and taste sense which may be related to formaldehyde exposure.

An allergist stated, ''I believe that Mrs. White's symptoms are caused and aggravated by exposure to urea-formaldehyde insulation.''

A pulmonologist found low grade and controlled hyperreactive airway disease, probably initiated by chronic exposure to urea-formaldehyde fumes.

Examination

Appearance.   Ms. White was dressed appropriately for the examination, and appeared her stated age.

Speech.   Ms. White's speech was clear and well formulated. No abnormalities such as slurring, mispronunciations, or stutters were present.

Orientation.   Ms. White was oriented to time, place, and to the examiner's role.

Test-taking Behavior.   Ms. White was very cooperative during the examination, but was visibly discouraged at times. She required extra emotional support during the examination. After the interview, Ms. White was observed crying in the waiting room and stated that "It is tough remembering how I used to be and what I have lost." During the afternoon testing, Ms. White had difficulty breathing and had to break to take medication. The testing took approximately 8 hours.

Test Results and Interpretation

Wechsler Adult Intelligence Scale, Revised: WAIS-R

	Scaled Scores Age-Adjusted	Percentile Rank	
Verbal Subscales			
Information	14	91	
Digit Span	13	84*	
Vocabulary	15	95	
Arithmetic	15	95	
Comprehension	15	95	
Similarities	13	84*	
Nonverbal Subscales			
Picture Completion	12	75*	
Picture Arrangement	14	91	
Block Design	15	95	
Object Assembly	12	75*	
Digit Symbol	12	75*	
Verbal IQ	126	96th	Superior
Performance IQ	119	90th	High Average
Full Scale IQ	125	95th	Superior

*Deficit

Previous Mental Function.   High school records indicated that Ms. White's IQ was in the very superior range (IQ average as listed by records as 135; a score as high as 144 was also found). Based on a premorbid IQ of 135, a scaled score of 17 (99th percentile) was used to interpret the WAIS-R. A cutoff scaled score of 13 (84th percentile) was used to demarcate deficit functioning.

Current Mental Function.   Full Scale IQ declined from a premorbid estimate average of 135 to 125, a decline of 10 points.

In the Verbal section of the WAIS-R, deficits were found in the Digit Span and Similarities Subtests, indicating deficits in *short-term memory* and *abstract thinking*.

In the Performance section of the WAIS-R, deficits were found by the Picture Completion, Object Assembly, and Digit Symbol Subtests, indicating deficits in *sequential thinking and the ability to see relationships between events, visuospatial and visuomotor abilities*, and *psychomotor reaction time*.

Benton Visual Retention Test.   This test assesses recent visual memory. Based upon Ms. White's premorbid IQ in the very superior range (135), 6 of 10 designs were expected correct, with 5 errors in reproduction. Ms. White remembered 8 designs, with 5 errors in reproduction. This performance was within normal range.

Wechsler Memory Scale: Logical Memory.   Based upon Ms. White's premorbid verbal IQ in the very superior range (135), it was expected that she would remember 34 elements upon immediate testing, and 19 elements upon delayed testing. Ms. White remembered 21 elements of the two stories upon immediate testing, which indicates deficiency ($p < .0005$) in *recent verbal memory* for logically related elements. Ms. White remembered 18 elements upon delayed testing, which is within the normal range when 21 elements are initially remembered.

The Embedded Figures Test.   This test evaluates the ability to detect visual figure-ground relationships. Ms. White detected all of the objects, within the normal range.

Grooved Pegboard Test.   This test evaluates manual dexterity. Time for completion was 76 seconds for the dominant hand, which is at approximately the 4th percentile, and 74 seconds for the nondominant hand, which is approximately at the 36th percentile, indicating a deficit in *manual dexterity*. Weakness in the left hand was noted during the NCV test.

Trailmaking Test.   This test evaluates visuomotor tracking, attention, and mental flexibility. Time for completing Part A was 40 seconds, which is approximately at the 8th percentile, a deficit in *visuomotor tracking and attention*. Time for completing Part B was 51 seconds, which is approximately at the 55 percentile, a deficit in *visuomotor tracking and mental flexibility*.

Paced Auditory Serial Addition Test.   This test evaluates *auditory information processing and tracking*. The results of this test indicate that Ms. White's performance was approximately at the 15th percentile, a deficit.

Controlled Oral Word Association Test.   This test evaluates verbal fluency. Ms. White's performance was measured at the 82nd percentile, a possible deficit in verbal fluency.

Gordon Diagnostic System.   This diagnostic device was used to assess vigilance, distractibility, and malingering.

Vigilance.   Within normal range.

Distractibility.   Probably abnormal.

Malingering.   Not indicated.

Summary of Deficits

Deficits were found in recent short-term memory, abstract thinking, sequential thinking and the ability to see relationships between events, visuospatial and visuomotor ability, psychomotor reaction time, recent auditory logical memory, manual dexterity, visuomotor tracking, attention, and mental flexibility, information processing and tracking, and distractibility.

Malingering Tests

Clinical Interview.   No evidence for malingering was found in the course of the interview. Ms. White's account of her exposure and condition remained constant and did not fluctuate under questioning. Her demeanor and affect were appropriate and credible.

Ungrouped Dot Counting.   This test is used to assess malingering. It requires the patient to count the number of dots drawn on cards. The cards are presented in random order; if the patient is not malingering, it will take more time to count the increasing number of dots. Malingering was not found.

Minnesota Multiphasic Personality Inventory. This test was used to assess malingering and psychological state. Malingering was not indicated on this test.

Gordon Diagnostic System. Results presented previously in this report.

Neurophysiologic Findings

Nerve conduction velocity (NCV) of the median motor, median sensory and sural (sensory) nerves were assessed. Median motor NCV was measured from elbow to wrist; median sensory NCV was measured from wrist to index finger; and sural NCV was measured from the calf to heel. See Appendix for the results.

Nerve conduction velocity test results indicated slowed nerve conduction and reduced amplitude of both sural nerves.

Conclusion

More likely than not, Ms. White showed the signs and symptoms of formaldehyde neurotoxicity. Epilepsy medication may also have affected her neuropsychologically. However, even after years of exposure to these medications, she was apparently quite active and efficient. After exposure to UFFI, she became disabled. I feel that this case provides some evidence of formaldehyde neurotoxicity.

APPENDIX
NERVE CONDUCTION VELOCITY

Name	Ellen White				
Age	57				
Side	Left		Side	Right	
Temp.	Arm	27.98	Temp.	Arm	27.88
Temp.	Leg	26.95	Temp.	Leg	25.55
	Velocity Meters/sec			Velocity Meters/sec	
Median	Motor	54.75	Median	Motor	56.00
Median	Sensory	43.95	Median	Sensory	38.16
Sural		23.97	Sural		16.88
	Amplitude (Motor in millivolts, sensory in microvolts)				
Median	Motor	21.20	Median	Motor	19.57
Median	Sensory	76.09	Median	Sensory	84.78
Sural		2.00	Sural		2.00

CASE REPORTS OF UREA FORMALDEHYDE FOAM INSULATION EXPOSURE OF A FAMILY
CASE 1: TONY VERDE

Tony Verde was a 39 year old male evaluated on February 14, 1987 for residual nervous system effects from exposure to urea formaldehyde foam insulation (UFFI).

Mr. Verde reported suffering from depression, mood changes, irritability, problems with memory and concentration, sleep problems, and headaches.

Exposure. In September 1977, UFFI was installed in the walls of the Verde home. The Verdes noticed an odor in their residence at that time. Over the next few years, the family experienced burning eyes, sore throats, excessive tiredness, amotivation, hypersensitivity to chemicals, depression, irritability, problems with memory and concentration, muscle weakness, numbness and confusion. By March 1982, the Verdes began to suspect that their health problems were caused by the UFFI. In October 1982, Mr. Verde removed the insulation from the walls.

Air Testing for Formaldehyde

Air tests performed by the State Department of Health Services in April, 1982, detected formaldehyde levels of .38 ppm in the room of Mr. Verde's son. Tests performed by Yerk Laboratories in the Verde residence in August 1982, found the following formaldehyde levels: downstairs living room, 0.11 ppm; upstairs rear corner bedroom, 0.08 ppm; upstairs living room, 0.10 ppm; upstairs kitchen, 0.09 ppm.

Field tests were performed by the State Department of Health Services in October 1982. Holes were drilled through the walls and UFFI was detected at different parts of home as follows: middle upstairs bedroom, 3 ppm; back upstairs kitchen, 10 ppm; back stairwell, 7 ppm; back stairs, 1 ppm; back lower stairway, 3 ppm; front downstairs living room, 4 ppm.

Additional tests performed by the State Department of Health Services in December 1982, detected formaldehyde as follows: downstairs living room, .12 ppm; upstairs living room, .12 ppm; Mr. Verde's son's room, .02 ppm; kitchen, .07 ppm. The UFFI had already been removed from all wall cavities. Apparently, the gas had been absorbed by wall and interior surfaces, as well as by furnishings, and continued to offgas, producing elevated levels of formaldehyde in the air.

Further testing in January 1983, found formaldehyde in the household air as follows: downstairs living room, 0.04 ppm; son's downstairs room, 0.06 ppm; (3) upstairs living room, 0.06 ppm. In March 1983, 0.05 ppm formaldehyde was still present in the son's downstairs room. See Appendix: Technical Factors of UFFI Installation, for further information.

Exposure Summary. The continuous elevated levels of formaldehyde gas show the persistence of this gas in the home environment. The earliest reading, taken five years after installation, showed levels that were a cause for concern (.08 to .38 ppm). The levels which had been present in earlier years must have been much higher.

Previous Medical History. The medical history reported by Mr. Verde revealed hospitalization and surgery for a broken leg. A severe cut on the right index finger was also reported. No other significant health problems before exposure were reported.

Test Results and Interpretation

Wechsler Adult Intelligence Scale, Revised: WAIS-R

	Scaled Scores Age-Adjusted	Percentile Rank	
Verbal Subscales			
Information	10	50	
Digit Span	11	63	
Vocabulary	10	50	
Arithmetic	10	50	
Comprehension	12	75	
Similarities	16	98	
Nonverbal Subscales			
Picture Completion	13	84	
Picture Arrangement	8	25	
Block Design	14	91	
Object Assembly	19	99.9	
Digit Symbol	14	91	
Verbal IQ	109	73rd	Average
Performance IQ	124	94th	Superior
Full Scale IQ	118	88th	High Average

Previous Mental Function. Based on school transcripts, it appeared that Mr. Verde was above average in mental ability before the exposure (and remains in the above average range, overall). An IQ of 118, high average (88th percentile), and a scaled score of 13 was used to interpret the test results. Scores below a scale score of 9, or the 37 percentile, were considered deficient.

Current Mental Function. In the Verbal section of the WAIS-R, a deficit was found in the Digit Span subtest, Digits Backward, indicating a deficit in *short-term memory*. Mr. Verde could only reliably remember three digits in the backwards direction.

In the Performance section of the WAIS-R, a deficit was indicated by the Picture Arrangement Subtest. The Picture Arrangement Subtest measured *sequential thinking and the ability to perceive relationships between events.*

Benton Visual Retention Test. This test assesses recent visual memory. Based upon Mr. Verde's estimated premorbid IQ in the high average range (118), 8 of 10 designs were expected to be correct, with 3 errors in reproduction. Mr. Verde remembered 7 designs, with 5 errors in reproduction. This performance is within normal range.

Wechsler Memory Scale: Logical Memory. Based upon Mr. Verde's current Verbal IQ of 109, it was expected that he would remember 23 elements upon immediate testing, and 16 elements upon delayed testing. Mr. Verde remembered only 17 elements of the two stories upon immediate testing, which indicates deficiency in *recent verbal memory* for logically related elements. In addition, Mr. Verde remembered only 9 elements upon delayed testing, indicating a deficit in *delayed verbal memory* for recently learned materials.

The Embedded Figures Test. This test evaluates the ability to detect visual figure-ground relationships. Mr. Verde detected 37 of the 40 objects, which is within normal range.

Grooved Pegboard Test. This test evaluates manual dexterity. Time for completion was 76 seconds for the dominant hand, which is approximately at the 25th percentile, and 62 seconds for the nondominant hand, which is approximately at the 40th percentile, indicating a deficit in *manual dexterity.*

Trailmaking Test. This test evaluates visuomotor tracking and attention. Time for completing Part A was 28 seconds, which is approximately at the 27th percentile, a deficit in *visuomotor tracking and attention.* Time for completing Part B was 63 seconds, which is approximately at the 30th percentile, a deficit in *mental flexibility.*

Paced Auditory Serial Addition Test. This test evaluates *auditory information processing and tracking.* The results of this test indicated that Mr. Verde was below the 1st percentile, a deficit.

Stroop Color and Word Test. This test evaluates the ease with which an individual can shift her/his perceptual set to conform to changing demands (cognitive flexibility). Mr. Verde's performance was deficit in Word Naming (21st percentile) and in Color Naming (33rd percentile). These test scores indicated deficiency in *reaction time.*

Controlled Oral Word Association Test. This test evaluates verbal fluency. Mr. Verde's performance was measured at the 60th percentile, within normal range.

Test Results

Deficits were found in recent short-term memory, recent and delayed auditory logical memory, manual dexterity, visuomotor tracking, auditory attention and information processing and tracking, mental flexibility, and reaction time.

Malingering Tests

Ungrouped Dot Counting. This examination requires the patient to count the number of dots drawn on cards. The cards are presented in a random order; if the patient is not malingering, it will take more time to count the increasing number of dots. Malingering was not found.

Symptom Endorsement Checklist. This test presents the opportunity for a patient to endorse symptoms that are highly unlikely for the ailment being investigated, which may raise the questions about the possibility of malingering. The response to these symptoms was negative. Malingering was not found.

Clinical Interview. No evidence for malingering was found in the course of the interview.

Neurophysiologic Findings

Nerve conduction velocity (NCV) of the median motor, median sensory and sural (sensory) nerves were assessed. Median motor NCV was measured from elbow to wrist; median sensory NCV was measured from wrist to index finger; and sural NCV was measured from the calf to heel.

Nerve conduction velocity test results were within normal range and are noncontributory.

Conclusion

Based upon the pattern of symptoms and neuropsychological findings in Mr. Verde and his wife (reported below), along with the history of exposure to elevated UFFI fumes, and onset of symptoms associated with UFFI exposure, I believe that this case provides evidence of formaldehyde neurotoxicity.

CASE 2: LINDA VERDE

Linda Verde was a 38 year old female evaluated on February 14, 1987 for residual nervous system effects from exposure to urea formaldehyde insulation.

Mrs. Verde reported suffering from depression, mood changes, irritability, personality changes, nervousness, confusion, problems with concentration and attention, trouble following conversation distractibility, sleep problems, fatigue, and unusually cold fingers and toes.

Previous Medical History.   Mrs. Verde reported suffering a broken arm, and rheumatic fever as a child. She reported an underactive thyroid condition for which she received medication in 1970–71. She also reported being hospitalized in 1974–75 for a miscarriage. When she was pregnant with her son Kenny she was diagnosed as being anemic. In addition, she reported a history of sinus and gastrointestinal problems.

Test Results and Interpretation

Wechsler Adult Intelligence Scale, Revised: WAIS-R

	Scaled Scores Age-Adjusted	Percentile Rank
Verbal Subscales		
Information	7	16
Digit Span	11	63
Vocabulary	8	25
Arithmetic	11	63
Comprehension	10	50
Similarities	9	37
Nonverbal Subscales		
Picture Completion	10	50
Picture Arrangement	7	16
Block Design	8	25
Object Assembly	9	37
Digit Symbol	11	63

Wechsler Adult Intelligence Scale, Revised: WAIS-R (Continued)

	Scaled Scores Age-Adjusted	Percentile Rank	
Verbal IQ	95	37th	Average
Performance IQ	92	30th	Average
Full Scale IQ	93	32nd	Average

Previous Mental Function. Based on school transcripts, Linda Verde obtained a Full Scale IQ of 106 when tested in the 8th grade. Using the formula of Barona et al. for estimating premorbid IQ, Mrs. Verde's IQ was calculated at 105, average (63rd percentile). An IQ of 105 and a scaled score of 11 was used to interpret the test results. Scores below a scale score of 7, or the 16th percentile, were considered deficient.

Current Mental Function. Overall, Mrs. Verde's intelligence decreased by approximately 13 IQ points, from the 63rd to the 32nd percentile.

In the Verbal section of the WAIS-R, a deficit was found in the Information Subtest, indicating a deficit in *general knowledge*. However, deficits on this test are not indicative of neurotoxicity.

In the Performance Section of the WAIS-R, a deficit was indicated by the Picture Arrangement Subtest. The Picture Arrangement Subtest measures *sequential thinking and the ability to see relationships between events*.

Benton Visual Retention Test. This test assesses recent visual memory. Based upon Mrs. Verde's estimated premorbid IQ in the average range (105), 7 of 10 designs were expected to be correct, with 4 errors in reproduction. Mrs. Verde remembered 6 designs, with 9 errors in reproduction. The error score is a strong indication of impairment of *recent visual memory*.

Wechsler Memory Scale: Logical Memory. Based upon Mrs. Verde's estimated premorbid verbal IQ of 105, it was expected that she would remember 23 elements upon immediate testing, and 13 elements upon delayed testing. Mrs. Verde remembered only 14 elements of the two stories upon immediate testing, which indicates deficiency in *recent verbal memory* for logically related elements. Mrs. Verde remembered 12 elements upon delayed testing.

The Embedded Figures Test. This test evaluates the ability to detect visual figure-ground relationships. Mrs. Verde detected 32 of the 40 objects, which is within the normal range.

Grooved Pegboard Test. This examination evaluates manual dexterity. Time for completion was 66 seconds for the dominant hand, which is approximately at the 18th percentile, and 73 seconds for the nondominant hand, which is approximately at the 18th percentile, indicating a borderline deficit in *manual dexterity*.

Trailmaking Test. This test evaluates visuomotor tracking and attention. Time for completing Part A was 28 seconds, which is approximately at the 16th percentile, a deficit in *visuomotor tracking and attention*. Time for completing Part B was 91 seconds, which is approximately at the 3rd percentile, a deficit in *mental flexibility*.

Paced Auditory Serial Addition Test. This test evaluates *auditory information processing and tracking*. The results of this test indicated that Mrs. Verde was below the 1st percentile, a deficit.

Stroop Color and Word Test. This examination evaluates the ease with which an individual can shift her/his perceptual set to conform to changing demands (cognitive flexibility). Mrs. Verde's performance was deficit in Color Naming (11th percentile). This test score indicates a deficiency in *reaction time*.

Controlled Oral Word Association Test. This test evaluates verbal fluency. Mrs. Verde's performance was measured at the 77th percentile, within the normal range.

Test Results

Deficits were found in recent short-term memory, recent visual memory, recent auditory logical memory, manual dexterity, visuomotor tracking, auditory attention and information processing and tracking, mental flexibility and reaction time.

Malingering Tests

Ungrouped Dot Counting. This test is used to assess malingering. It requires the patient to count the number of dots drawn on cards. The cards are presented in a random order; if the patient is not malingering, it takes more time to count the increasing number of dots. Malingering was not found.

Symptom Endorsement Checklist. This test is used to assess malingering. If the patient endorses symptoms that are highly unlikely for the ailment being investigated, it may raise a question about the possibility of malingering. The response to these symptoms was negative. Malingering was not found.

Clinical Interview. No evidence for malingering was found in the course of the interview.

Neurophysiologic Findings

Nerve conduction velocity (NCV) of the median motor, median sensory and sural (sensory) nerves were assessed. Median motor NCV was measured from elbow to wrist; median sensory NCV was measured from wrist to index finger; and sural NCV was measured from the calf to the heel. See appendix for results.

Nerve conduction velocity test results indicated reduced amplitude in the left median motor nerve, and both sural nerves. Slowing of the right median sensory nerve was found, and the left median sensory nerve was within the slow range.

Conclusion

Based upon the pattern of symptoms and neuropsychological findings in Mrs. Verde and her husband, the history of exposure to elevated UFFI fumes, and the onset of symptoms associated with UFFI exposure, I believe that this case provided evidence of formaldehyde neurotoxicity.

APPENDIX
NERVE CONDUCTION VELOCITY, TONY VERDE

Age	39				
Side	Left		Side	Right	
Temp.	Arm	25.98	Temp.	Arm	25.70
Temp.	Leg	25.55	Temp.	Leg	25.45
	Velocity Meters/sec			Velocity Meters/sec	
Median	Motor	50.19	Median	Motor	50.38
Median	Sensory	39.27	Median	Sensory	37.93
Sural		35.00	Sural		34.72
	Amplitude (Motor in millivolts, sensory in microvolts)				
Median	Motor	15.76	Median	Motor	21.74
Median	Sensory	60.87	Median	Sensory	63.04
Sural		28.26	Sural		39.13

APPENDIX
NERVE CONDUCTION VELOCITY, LINDA VERDE

Age	38				
Side	Left		Side	Right	
Temp.	Arm	29.23	Temp.	Arm	29.68
Temp.	Leg	31.45	Temp.	Leg	30.85
	Velocity Meters/sec			Velocity Meters/sec	
Median	Motor	57.14	Median	Motor	56.22
Median	Sensory	37.05	Median	Sensory	35.91
Sural		44.57	Sural		45.58
	Amplitude (Motor in millivolts, sensory in microvolts)				
Median	Motor	6.52	Median	Motor	11.96
Median	Sensory	47.83	Median	Sensory	43.48
Sural		19.57	Sural		13.04

APPENDIX
TECHNICAL FACTORS OF UFFI INSTALLATION

Insulating foams are cellular materials that contain bubbles of gas. Various types can be made, ranging from rigid types to those very soft in texture. Flexible foams are used extensively in cushioning, while rigid foams are best known for their thermal insulation. Generally, the rigid foams are closed cells (gas totally enclosed by cell walls) and flexible systems have open cells. The cells have to be open to have high flexibility so that air can escape on compression (Driver, 1979).

Urea foams are reaction products of urea and formaldehyde. Commercial systems are used for foaming areas such as walls, floors, and roofs. Urea foams are applied using a two-component machine. The foam is fully expanded, like shaving cream, when it leaves the nozzle. This feature allows the foam to be applied in wall cavities without damaging or distorting the structure. Flame resistance of urea foams is inherently good. Thermal conductivity is not as good as in fluorocarbon-blown urethanes because the cell structure in urea foams is mostly open. Moisture and elevated temperatures have been known to break down urea foams, producing an objectionable formaldehyde odor; shrinkage has also been a problem (Driver, 1979).

Although the amount and duration of formaldehyde release can vary, laboratory tests have shown that every foam insulation product tested in the United States releases a measurable amount of formaldehyde gas and that the release continues for a prolonged period of time. The Consumer Product Safety Commission is not aware of any brand or type of the product that does not release some formaldehyde gas after it is installed. After installation, the product may continue to release formaldehyde gas for years. Formaldehyde emissions from UFFI would tend to be higher during hot and humid periods (CPSC, 1982).

The amount of formaldehyde gas emitted by urea formaldehyde insulation is dependent upon a number of factors, ranging from the expertise of the installer to an excess of formaldehyde in the resin; an excess of catalyst in the foaming agent; improper ratio of resin to foaming agent; excess amount of foaming agent; and problems with humidity. As formation of the foam insulation is done on the work site, exacting standards are difficult to ensure.

Environmental factors affecting offgassing include temperature, season, and humidity. Heat from a hot summer day or heat from a furnace in winter will increase the degassing of the foam insulation. Not only ambient conditions within the home, but also seasonal temperature and humidity fluctuations in the atmosphere will affect the rate of "offgassing." Chemical factors affecting offgassing; the urea formaldehyde bond is constantly broken with increasing temperature and the addition of moisture. As a result, all urea foams "offgass" formaldehyde to some degree regardless of the method of installation (Garry et al., 1980).

REFERENCES

CPSC. 1982. Consumer Product Safety Commission: Ban of Urea Formaldehyde Foam Insulation, Withdrawal of Proposed Information Labeling Rule, and Denial of Petition to Issue a Standard. *Federal Register*. Volume 47, No. 64.

Driver, Walter E. 1979. *Plastics Chemistry and Technology*. Van Nostrand Reinhold: New York, NY, pp. 87–105.

Garry, Vincent F.; Oatman, Laura; Pleus, Richard; and Gray, David. 1980. *Formaldehyde in the Home, Some Environmental Disease Perspectives*. Minnesota Dept. of Health. pp. 107–111.

6
NEUROTOXICITY OF SELECTED SUBSTANCES

This chapter includes neurotoxicity reports for selected neurotoxic substances: ammonia, BTX (benzene, toluene, and xylene), carbon monoxide, chlordane, formaldehyde, gasoline, organic lead, cadmium, manganse, organic mercury, organophosphorous pesticides, PCB, and also radiation. The chemicals were selected to represent the range of substances that can be neurotoxic. Each of the substances were involved in neurotoxicity cases that I have researched.

THE NEUROTOXICITY OF AMMONIA

Chemistry of Ammonia

Ammonia (NH_3) is a colorless, suffocating, combustible gas with a penetrating, pungent odor. Ammonia is produced by synthesis, using nitrogen from the atmosphere (Haber-Bosch Process). It is a high-tonnage chemical used in the manufacture of sodium carbonate and bicarbonate (Solvay Process), hydrogen cyanide, nitric acid, ammonium nitrate, and acrylonitrile. Ammonia is a component of fertilizers and explosives, a refrigerant used for large-scale fish and food preservation, a catalyst, and a stabilizer of rubber latex. It has some medicinal use in smelling salts and aromatic spirits. When dissolved in water at concentrations of up to 30%, it forms ammonium hydroxide (NH_4OH) (Clayton and Clayton, 1981; Gosselin et al., 1984, Windholtz et al., 1983).

Ammonium hydroxide (ammonia water, aqua ammonia, "Spirit of Hartshorn") is a colorless liquid with an intense, pungent suffocating odor and an acrid taste. It is used as a detergent and a household cleaning agent, as a bleaching agent in calico printing and for extracting plant colors and alkaloids. Ammonium hydroxide is also used in the manufacturing of aluminum salts and azo and aniline dyes (Clayton and Clayton, 1981; Gosselin et al., 1984, Windholtz et al., 1983).

Toxicity of Ammonia

Ammonia vapor is a severe irritant of the eyes (especially the cornea), the respiratory tract, and the skin. It may cause burning and tearing of the eyes, runny noise, coughing, and chest pain. Exposure of the eyes to high gas concentrations can produce temporary blindness and severe eye damage. Exposure of the skin to high concentrations of the gas can cause burning and blistering of the skin. Inhalation of concentrations of 2500 to 6500 ppm causes dyspnea (difficult or painful breathing), bronchospasm, chest pain and pulmonary edema, which may be fatal (Mackinson et al. 1981). A major consequence of inhalation may be ammonia intoxication with symptoms of edema, spasm of the glottis, slurred speech, blurred vision, and in severe cases, death. These symptoms resemble those of the syndrome of hepatic coma, which occurs when blood, and presumably, brain ammonia levels are elevated (Harper et al., 1979).

Once absorbed, ammonia is converted to the ammonium ion as the hydroxide and to salts, especially as carbonates. Ammonium salts are converted to urea to maintain an isotonic system (Clayton and Clayton, 1981). Excess ammonium ions which remain and concentrate in the blood result in a condition called hyperammonemia.

Ammonia has a toxic action on the central nervous system and can produce encephalopathy (brain disease). Abnormalities of ammonia metabolism are most frequently thought to cause the pathogenesis of hepatic encephalopathy. Evidence in favor of ammonia as the principal toxin in most patients suffering from hepatic encephalopathy includes: (1) an elevated arterial or cerebrospinal fluid ammonia in the majority of patients with this disorder; (2) induction of hepatic encephalopathy in susceptible patients by administration of ammonium salts; (3) relief of the syndrome following therapy directed towards reduction of blood ammonia; and (4) presence of hepatic encephalopathy in children with genetically determined deficiencies of the enzymes of the Krebs-Henseleit cycle, leading to hyperammonemia (Harvey et al., 1984).

Ammonia is known to affect the function of the neurons in several ways:

1. Ammonia can depolarize neurons by substituting for K^+. This substitution initially increases neuronal excitability, but eventually causes a depolarizing block.
2. Ammonia can affect synaptic transmission at a presynaptic site, because the inhibition of glutaminase by ammonia can decrease the availability of glutamate, aspartate, and GABA as synaptic transmitters.
3. Ammonia can affect postsynaptic inhibition and decrease the hyperpolarizing action of the postsynaptic inhibition (Raabe and Lin, 1984).

The current OSHA (Occupational Safety and Health Administration, of the U.S. Department of Labor) standard for ammonia is 50 parts of ammonia per million parts of air (ppm) averaged over an eight hour work shift. This may also be expressed as 35 milligrams of ammonia per cubic meter of air (mg/m^3). NIOSH (National Institute of Occupational Safety and Health, U.S. Department of Health and Human Services) has recommended that the permissible exposure limit be changed to a ceiling of 50 ppm (35 mg/m^3) averaged over a five minute period (Harvey et al, 1984).

Motor Neuron Disease

Motor neuron disease (MND) is a condition characterized by progressive weakness and atrophy of the skeletal muscles. It can manifest itself in several different forms, multiple sclerosis and amyotrophic lateral sclerosis being examples. Hyperammonemia can cause motor neuron dysfunction as exhibited in one of five syndromes (Shih, 1978):

1. Carbamoyl phosphate synthetase deficiency (congenital hyperammonemia type I): degeneration of the brainstem, hypomyelination (myelin is the fatty tissue, which forms the insulating sheath that surrounds certain nerve fibers) and loss of neurons.
2. Ornithine carbamoyl transferase deficiency (congenital hyperammonemia type II): overall swelling of brain tissue with dilated ventricles, and destruction of cerebral cortex tissue.
3. Citrullinemia: microscopic brain lesions including degeneration of nerve cell myelin and enlarged glial cells.
4. Argininosuccinic aciduria: spongy alteration of white and gray matter, deficiency in myelinization and degeneration of myelin sheaths.
5. Hyperargininemia: cerebral atrophy and enlarged ventricles.

High levels of ammonia have been described at the site of the anterior horn spinal cord tissue from patients who have died of MND. The amount of ammonia was found to bear a direct relationship to the severity of the disease process. This suggests that ammonia can also contribute directly to motor neuron dysfunction (Patten et al., 1982).

REFERENCES

Clayton, G. D. and Clayton, F. E. 1981. *Patty's Industrial Hygiene and Toxicology*, 3rd Edition. John Wiley & Sons: New York, NY, pp. 3045–3052.

Gosselin, R. E., Smith, R. P., and Hodge, H. C. 1984. *Clinical Toxicology of Commercial Products*. 5th Edition. Williams & Wilkins: Baltimore, Section III, pp. 21–26.

Harper, H. A., Mayes, P. A., Rodwell, V. W. 1979. *Review of Physiological Chemistry*. 17th Edition. Lange Medical Publications: Los Altos, CA, p. 400.

Harvey, A. M., Johns, R. J., McKusick, V. A., Owens, A. H., Jr., and Ross, R. S. (Eds.) 1984. *The Principles and Practice of Medicine*. 21st Edition. Appleton-Century-Crofts: Norwalk, CT, pp. 734–745.

Mackinson, F. and Partridge, L. J. Jr. (Eds.) 1981. *Occupational Health Guidelines for Chemical Hazards*, DHHS (NIOSH) Publication, No. 81-123.

Patten, B. M., Kurlander, H. M., and Evans, B. 1982. Free amino acid concentrations in spinal tissue from patients dying of motor neuron disease, *Acta Neurol. Scandinav.* 66:594–599.

Raabe, W. and Lin, S. 1984. Ammonia, Postsynaptic Inhibition and CNS-Energy State. *Brain Research*, 303:67–76.

Shih, V. E. 1978. Urea Cycle Disorders and Other Congenital Hyperammonemic Syndromes. *The Metabolic Basis of Inherited Disease*. 4th Edition. Stanbury, Wyngaarten, Fredrickson, (Eds.). McGraw-Hill: New York, NY, pp. 362–386.

Windholz, M., Badavari, S., Blumetti, R., and Otterbein, E. S. (Eds.) 1983. *The Merk Index*. 10th Edition. Merck & Co.: Rahway, NJ, p. 74.

ACUTE TOXICITY AND CHRONIC TOXICITY OF BENZENE AND BTX

Benzene is rated very toxic. Between 1 teaspoon and 1 ounce of benzene would be fatal to the average person (Gosselin et al., 1984).

Benzene is a clear, colorless liquid with a characteristic pleasant odor at low concentrations, and a disagreeable odor at higher concentrations. It is the simplest aromatic compound known. Benzene has been one of the most important industrial chemicals. However, because of its toxicity, benzene has been replaced in many applications by other solvents, such as toluene (Clayton and Clayton, 1981).

BTX consists of benzene, toluene, and xylene. BTX is added to gasoline to increase its octane rating, and has gained in usage as the gasoline additive lead is phased out. See gasoline described later in this chapter.

Acute Toxicity — Oral and Dermal

Ingestion of 9 to 12 grams of benzene has caused staggering gait, vomiting, somnolence, shallow/rapid pulse, loss of consciousness, and later delirium, with subsequent chemical pneumonitis, serious collapse due to initial stimulation, then abrupt CNS depression. Generally, at moderate concentrations, symptoms are dizziness, excitation, and pallor, followed by flushing, weakness, headache, breathlessness, and constriction of the chest. Visual disturbances and convulsions are frequent symptoms. At higher concentrations the symptoms are excitement and euphoria, which quite suddenly change to weariness, fatigue, and sleepiness, followed by coma and death (Clayton and Clayton, 1981).

Dermal absorption is slower than absorption through the mucous membranes.

Acute Toxicity — Inhalation

In acute respiratory exposures, benzene, toluene, and xylene produce similar toxic reactions, consisting primarily of local irritation of the respiratory tract, and CNS excitation and depression. The symptoms resemble those of ethyl alcohol inebriation with euphoria and all stages of CNS depression up to anesthesia and respiratory arrest. The signs of CNS depression such as emotional instability, impaired motor coordination, slurred speech, ataxia (loss of the power of muscular coordination), nystagmus (rhythmical oscillation of the eyeballs), stupor, and coma, may be punctuated by episodes of neuroirritability, for which the physiologic basis is not well understood. Aromatic hydrocarbons (chemicals with one or more benzene rings) induce states of unconsciousness which are accompanied by tremors, motor restlessness, hypertonia (extreme restlessness or tossing about from side to side) and generally hyperactive reflexes, while the aliphatic petroleum hydrocarbons (straight or branched chains of carbon atoms, rather than a ring, to which hydrogen atoms are attached), is associated with deep coma and depressed reflexes (Gosselin et al, 1984).

When inhaled at 25 ppm, benzene may result in no obvious effect, but at 50 to 150 ppm it produces headache, lassitude, and weariness, and at 500 ppm causes more exaggerated symptoms; 3,000 ppm may be tolerated for 0.5 to 1.0 hr; 7,500 ppm may result in toxic signs in 0.5 to 1.0 hr; and 20,000 ppm may be fatal if inhaled for 5 to 10 minutes (Clayton and Clayton, 1981). According to one study, the fatal benzene level is 19,000 to 20,000 ppm for 5 to 10 minutes; 7,500 ppm for 30 minutes is dangerous to life; 1,500 ppm for 60 minutes produces serious symptoms of illness; and 50 to 150 ppm for five hours produces headache, lassitude and weakness (Gerarde, 1960).

Chronic Toxicity — Inhalation

Chronic inhalation of benzene on a lower-level repeated basis appears to be related to a number of pathological conditions. The levels which produce effects vary widely with individuals. Contributing factors are poor nutrition, certain immunologic tendencies, and consumption of alcohol or drugs

Some symptoms include headaches, dizziness, fatigue, dyspnea, visual disturbances, and vague symptoms that are not usually connected with benzene poisoning. Signs also include fatigue, vertigo, pallor, visual disturbances, and loss of consciousness (Clayton and Clayton, 1981).

The following specific symptoms have been reported: fatigue, dizziness, dryness of mucous membranes, hemorrhaging, nausea or vomiting, lethargy, weakness, epistaxis (nosebleeds), loss of appetite, shortness of breath, dizziness, hematopathy, thrombocytopenia (abnormally small number of platelets), lymphatic effects, aplastic anemia (defective regeneration of leukocytes and hemoglobin caused by aplastic or unregenerative bone marrow), leukopenia (abnormally low numbers of white blood cells) and chromosomal aberrations. Low, intermittent exposure results in very subtle hematopoietic changes; moderate to high exposures affect enzyme synthesis, causing anemias; and high exposures produce irreversible blood dyscrasias (permanent abnormal cellular elements in the blood) (Clayton and Clayton, 1981).

Because of its insidious onset and the large numbers of people exposed to benzene, chronic benzene poisoning is of far greater toxicologic significance than is acute poisoning. In most cases, chronic benzene poisoning has followed repeated exposures to unsafe air levels of benzene vapor over the course of months or years. Clinical manifestations of chronic benzene poisoning tend to be insidious in onset, and most recorded causes have been well advanced at the time of diagnosis (Finkel, 1983).

REFERENCES

Gosselin, R. E., Smith, R. P., Hodge, H. C. 1984. *Clinical Toxicology of Commercial Products* (5th Ed.), Section III., Baltimore: Williams & Wilkins. pp. 397–404.

Clayton, G. D. and Clayton, F. E. 1981. *Patty's Industrial Hygiene and Toxicology*, 3rd Ed. Vol. 2B. New York: John Wiley & Sons. pp. 3260–3283.

Gerarde, H. W. 1960, *Toxicology and Biochemistry of Aromatic Hydrocarbons*, New York: Elsevier. Found in *Drinking Water Criteria*, Document for Benzene (Final Draft) (April, 1985). US EPA, Washington, DC.

Finkel, A. J. 1983, *Hamilton and Hardy's Industrial Toxicology*. 4th Ed. Boston: John Wright, PSG Inc. pp. 245–248.

ACUTE TOXICITY AND CHRONIC TOXICITY OF TOLUENE

Acute Toxicity—Inhalation

The primary effect of toluene is on the central nervous system (CNS). The effect may be depressant or excitatory, with euphoria in the induction phase followed by disorientation, tremulousness, hallucinations, ataxia, convulsions, and coma. Acute controlled and occupational exposures to toluene in the range of 200 to 1500 ppm caused dose-related CNS effects. Acute exposure to high levels of toluene, e.g., 10,000 ppm or higher, for several minutes during industrial accidents was characterized by initial CNS excitative effects (e.g., exhilaration, euphoria, hallucinations) followed by progressive impairment of consciousness, eventually resulting in seizures and coma. Single, short-term exposures to toluene (200 ppm for 8 hours) have reportedly caused transient eye and respiratory tract irritation, with lachrymation at 400 ppm (WHO, 1985).

Experimental exposures of up to 800 ppm toluene have produced acute dose-related CNS alterations. In single 8-hour exposures, three subjects were subjected to concentrations of toluene that ranged from 50–800 ppm in an exposure chamber. A maximum of two exposures per week were conducted; a total of 22 exposures were performed over an 8 week period. Subjective complaints of fatigue, muscular weakness, confusion, and impaired coordination were reported at levels of 200 ppm. These effects increased in severity with increases in toluene concentration, until at 800 ppm the subjects experienced severe fatigue, pronounced nausea, mental confusion, considerable incoordination and staggering gait, strongly impaired pupillary light reflex, and after-effects (muscular fatigue, nervousness, and insomnia) that lasted for several days (USEPA, 1983).

Short-term experimental exposures to toluene have also elicited decreases in reaction time and reduction in perceptual speed. In a test, 23 Japanese subjects given single exposures to 200 ppm toluene showed increased eye-to-hand time (USEPA, 1983).

In a more extensive study, 12 male subjects were exposed to 100, 300, 500, or 700 ppm toluene (via breathing valve and mouthpiece) during successive 20 minute exposure periods and their performance was measured on four tests of perceptual speed and reaction time. Results of the study showed both reaction time and perceptual speed were impaired during exposure to toluene. A significant effect on reaction time was noted with exposure to 300 ppm. Subject reaction time was further impaired at higher levels of exposure (500 and 700 ppm), but no impairment was noted for exposure to 100 ppm (USEPA, 1983).

Occupational exposure to 43 to 254 ppm toluene changed mood and caused difficulties in concentration and coordination in such a manner that the disturbances could be expected to diminish the ability to drive a car (Snyder, 1987).

Transient abnormalities of hepatic enzyme activities have been found in abusers of toluene mixtures. Occasional reports of renal damage in glue-sniffers characterized by a form of distal tubular acidosis have been reported.

Narcosis is the primary result of acute toluene exposure at high concentrations. Data on toluene abuse suffer from lack of experimental control and lack of documentation of actual exposure levels and toxicant purity, but provide information about very high level exposures. In case studies, a large variety of symptoms are reported, but the most common findings with long sniffing histories are motor weakness, intention tremor ataxia, and in one case, evidence of cerebral atrophy (USEPA 1983).

Acute Toxicity—Ingestion

Between one teaspoon and one ounce of toluene taken orally would be fatal to the average person (Gosselin, et al, 1984). Oral absorption appears to occur more slowly than that through the respiratory tract (WHO, 1985).

Acute Toxicity—Dermal

In human volunteer studies, absorption through the skin occurred following exposure to liquid toluene (rate of absorption 14 to 23 mg/cm^2 per hour) and, to a much lesser extent, following exposure to saturated aqueous solutions (rate of absorption 0.16 to .6 mg/cm² per hour). A maximum toluene concentration in the blood of 0.17 mg/l was found when the skin of volunteers was immersed in liquid toluene for 30 minutes (WHO, 1985).

Chronic Toxicity—Inhalation

Repeated occupational exposures to toluene over a period of years at levels of 200 to 400 ppm have resulted in some evidence of neurological effects (WHO, 1985).

Toluene-containing mixtures have been implicated in the causation of peripheral neuropathy, but in most cases, known neurotoxins such as n-hexane or methyl ethyl ketone have been present, and the role of toluene is not clear (WHO, 1985).

Irreversible neurological sequelae, such as encephalopathy, optic atrophy, and equilibrium disorders have been described in adult chronic toluene abusers. Toluene inhalation was reported to be an important cause of encephalopathy in children aged 8 to 14 years and may lead to permanent neurological damage (WHO, 1985).

The following effects were reported by 200 of 1,000 workers who showed symptoms due to commercial toluene exposure that were severe enough to seek examination at a hospital. The workers had been exposed daily to toluene concentrations ranging from 50 to 1500 ppm for periods of 1 to 3 weeks (WHO, 1985).

With an exposure of 50 to 200 ppm (approximately 60% of the patients): headache, lassitude, and loss of appetite.

With an exposure of 200 to 500 ppm (approximately 30% of the patients): headache, nausea, anorexia, lassitude, slight but definite impairment of coordination and reaction time, and momentary loss of memory.

With an exposure of 500 to 1500 ppm (approximately 10% of the patients): nausea, headache, dizziness, anorexia, palpitation, and extreme weakness; loss of coordination was pronounced and reaction time was definitely impaired.

Residual effects caused by cerebellar and cerebral dysfunction have been observed in a number of persons who had abused toluene or solvent mixtures containing toluene over a period of years. Clinical signs in these individuals include ataxia, intention tremors, nystagmus, equilibrium disorders, impairment of speech and hearing, reduced vision, disturbance of concentration and

memory, and psychosis. Prolonged toluene abuse has led to permanent encephalopathy and brain atrophy as revealed by EEG and neuroradiological changes
(USEPA, 1983).

In a Japanese study of 38 female shoemakers (mean age 20.7 ± 5.2 years)
exposed to a glue containing mainly toluene for an average duration of 3 years
and 4 months, the average toluene concentration in the air varied with the time
of year from 60 to 100 ppm (range 15 to 200 ppm). Results of neurological
and muscular function tests repeatedly showed abnormal tendon reflexes, reduced grasping power of the dominant hand, and decreased finger tapping tempo
in the exposed workers relative to a group of 16 unexposed control women. A
significant decrease in finger agility was also noted in the exposed shoemakers;
agility of the finger was estimated by measuring the time needed to move 25
"bulbs" using glass chopsticks (USEPA, 1983).

Electroneuromyographic measurements were made on 59 toluene-exposed car
painters and 53 referents with a similar age distribution for an indication of
possible peripheral neurotoxic effect from chronic toluene exposure. Maximum
motor conduction velocity (MCV), conduction velocity of the slower motor
fibers (CVSF), maximal sensory conduction velocity (SCV), and motor distal
latencies were recorded from nerves in the upper and lower extremities (median,
ulnar, deep peroneal, posterior tibial, and sural nerves). Results of these measurements showed that the mean conduction velocities and motor distal latencies
of the painters were almost identical to those recorded for the unexposed control
group. In several instances, however, individual nerve conduction velocities
were found to be slower than the normal historical value. When the conduction
velocities of the study group were compared with the historical values, abnormally slow MCVs, SCVs and/or prolonged motor distal latencies were found
in 12 of the 59 painters, but in none of the 53 controls (USEPA, 1983).

Peripheral biopsies of radial cutaneous nerves showed distention of axons,
thinning of the myelin sheath, widening of the nodes of Ranvier, and axonal
degeneration of large diameter fibers in the sural nerve in workers occupation-
ally exposed to toluene (WHO, 1985).

The toxicity of xylene is similar to the toxicity of toluene, and will not be
discussed here.

REFERENCES

WHO, *Environmental Health Criteria 52: Toluene.* 1985. World Health Organization,
   International Programme on Chemical Safety, Geneva, Switzerland.
USEPA. Health Assessment Document for Toluene: Final Report. 1983. PB84-100056.
Snyder, R. (Ed.) 1987. *Ethel Browning's Toxicity and Metabolism of Industrial Sol-
   vents*, (2nd Ed.), Vol. I.
Gosselin, R. E., Smith, R. P., and Hodge, H. C. 1984. *Clinical Toxicology of Com-
   mercial Products*, (5th Ed.), Section III, p. 153.

CARBON MONOXIDE TOXICITY

Mechanisms of Carbon Monoxide Toxicity. Carbon monoxide combines with hemoglobin. Its affinity for hemoglobin is 250 to 260 times that of oxygen. Therefore it binds with hemoglobin and leads to a lack of oxygen in blood. A level of 0.4% can be fatal after 1 hour.

Patients who survive acute exposure are at risk of disability or death from the effects of carbon monoxide on the central nervous system. Poisoning may result in lethal cerebral edema as a consequence of cell death that is caused by hypoxia and interference with cellular respiration. Central nervous system disorders due to delayed deterioration have long been recognized as a sequelae of carbon monoxide poisoning. Delayed deterioration is also associated with diffuse demyelinization. A three-year follow-up of patients with carbon monoxide poisoning revealed that 11% suffered neuropsychiatric disturbances, the most common being irritability, impulsiveness, mood changes, violence, and verbal aggressiveness. Personality changes, cognitive abnormalities, and neurologic abnormalities were common in patients with decreased levels of consciousness at the time of admission to hospital (Dolan, 1985).

Carbon monoxide affects the body in three ways:

1. Inhibition of oxygen transport. Carbon monoxide competes with oxygen for binding sites on hemoglobin. Normally oxygen joins with hemoglobin to form oxyhemoglobin. In carbon monoxide poisoning, carboxyhemoglobin (HbCO) is produced instead. Carboxyhemoglobin is the major form of carbon monoxide transport in the body. The net effect of this preferential binding of carbon monoxide to hemoglobin is a reduction of oxygen content of blood and tissue resulting in generalized hypoxia.
2. Effect of carbon monoxide on oxygen delivery. Carboxyhemoglobin results in hemoglobin binding more tightly to the oxygen that is available. As a result, tissue hypoxia is greater than one would expect from simply reducing the level of functioning hemoglobin.
3. Effect of carbon monoxide on oxygen utilized by the tissues. Carbon monoxide directly inhibits the action of cytochrome oxydase systems. These enzyme systems are iron-containing proteins and thus are directly bound by carbon monoxide. The cytochrome oxidase system is also the site of great metabolic activity. Thus organs with the highest metabolic rate, e.g., heart and CNS, are affected the most by carbon monoxide poisoning. The binding of carbon monoxide to the cytochrome oxidase system inhibits cellular respiration by displacing oxygen (Myers, 1985).

Tests of arterial blood gas levels include:

1. pH: Low pH, less than 7.40, usually represents metabolic acidosis secondary to tissue hypoxia. Metabolic acidosis from CO poisoning is associated with poor prognosis.
2. PAO_2: This test is a measure of O_2 dissolved in the blood and thus is not directly affected by CO exposure; it may, in fact, be elevated if the patient is hyperventilating or receiving supplemental O_2.
3. $PACO_2$: Normal or elevated $PACO_2$ (greater than 40 mm Hg) in the presence of metabolic acidosis suggests respiratory depression or failure. A carboxyhemoglobin percentage in blood of 50% corresponds with greater than 50 ppm carbon monoxide in alveolar air (Meyers, 1985).

Smith and Brandon (1973) evaluated 74 survivors of acute carbon monoxide poisoning over a three-year period. In 8 patients, gross neuropsychiatric damage was directly attributable to the poisoning. Three patients committed suicide, and 8 died from other causes. Of the 63 patients alive at follow-up, 8 showed an improvement and 21 (33%) a deterioration of personality after poisoning, and 27 (43%) showed a subsequent impairment of memory. Deterioration of personality and memory impairment were highly correlated. The level of consciousness on admission to hospital in the acute phase of poisoning correlated significantly with the development of gross neuropsychiatric sequelae.

Ginsberg (1979) reported a delayed neurological deterioration following hypoxia. He reviewed a number of case studies of delayed post-hypoxic deterioration, with reference to the clinical manifestations, the neuropathological findings, and delayed neurological deterioration in the absence of white matter pathology.

Ginsberg and Romano (1976) reviewed carbon monoxide encephalopathy. A review of the literature revealed that 15 to 40% of survivors of carbon monoxide poisoning developed neuropsychiatric symptoms, often following a period of apparent recovery. Patients often have negative neurological and psychiatric examinations within several days after their original exposure and are either discharged from the hospital or allowed to become ambulatory. The patient usually does well for between 2 to 21 days and then can develop the whole spectrum of neuropsychiatric signs and symptoms. Deterioration may either progress to coma or death or become arrested at any point. Some patients have a second recovery period which can lead to full health. There is no way to distinguish those patients who will recover from those who will relapse. In their article, the authors found that bedrest for 2 to 4 weeks seemed necessary to avoid delayed onset of neuropsychiatric symptoms. Although the exact etiology of this delayed onset is not known, the authors found a clear correlation between the onset of delayed symptoms and increased patient activity. They also stated that tranquilizing drugs that decrease REM sleep should be avoided.

Georgemiller and Baumchen (1987) reported two cases of amnestic syndrome following acute carbon monoxide intoxication. Both patients displayed severe recent and remote memory impairment, with five factors in common: (1) rapid forgetting; (2) normal short-term memory; (3) responsiveness to recognition probes; (4) responsiveness to retrieval cues; and (5) increased proactive interference.

REFERENCES

Dolan, M. C. 1985. Carbon monoxide poisoning. *Can. Med. Assoc. J.* 133:393–99.

Georgemiller, R. J., and Baumchen, H. A. 1987. Neuropsychological assessment of amnestic syndrome following acute carbon monoxide intoxication. Paper presented at the National Academy of Neuropsychologists Annual Meeting, Chicago, October 1987.

Ginsberg, M. D. 1979. Delayed neurological deterioration following hypoxia. *Advances in Neurology* 26:21–45.

Ginsberg, R., and Romano, J. 1976. Carbon monoxide encephalopathy: Need for appropriate treatment. *Am. J. Psychiat.* 133:(3) 317–20.

Myers, R. A. M. 1985. Carbon monoxide poisoning. In *Environmental Emergencies*, R. N. Nelson, D. A. Rund and M. D. Keller, Editors. W. B. Saunders Company: Philadelphia.

Smith, S. J., and Brandon, S. 1973. Morbidity from acute carbon monoxide poisoning at three year follow-up. *Brit. Med. J.* 1:318–321.

THE TOXICITY OF CHLORDANE AND HEPTACHLOR

Chlordane and heptachlor are cyclodiene pesticides. The symptoms of toxicity in man are similar for the cyclodiene insecticides, so a separate discussion by compounds is unnecessary (Ecobichon and Joy, 1982). In this section, the term chlordane will refer to both chlordane and heptachlor except where noted.

Chlordane is a well-known chemical product that can be hazardous to human health. It is rated very toxic (between 1 tsp to 1 ounce is the probable oral lethal dose for a 150 lb human). The acute oral LD50 in rats has been reported variously as 250 and 590 mg/kg (Gosselin et al., 1984).

Chlordane is a stimulant of the central nervous system. It has been estimated that the fatal oral dose for an adult human lies somewhere between 6 and 60 grams.

Chronic poisoning in animals produces degenerative changes in the liver, kidney, lungs, intestines, and heart. Chlordane is an established carcinogen in mouse liver. Research reports have implicated chlordane as a cause of leukemia and neuroblastoma (Gosselin et al., 1984).

The earliest signs of chlordane poisoning are increased sensitivity to stimuli due to hyperexcitability of the central nervous system, generalized hyperactive reflexes, muscle twitching, tremor, incordination, ataxia, and clonic convulsions with or without coma. Cycles of excitement and depression may be repeated several times (Gosselin et al., 1984).

The Neurotoxicity of Chlordane

Unfortunately, chlordane and other insecticides have been widely used without adequate safety testing prior to sale. The GAO has concluded that the risks of most pesticides remain uncertain, as they have not been fully tested and evaluated in accordance with current testing requirements (GAO, 1986a). Instead of a systematic testing program, the product safety is evaluated on an ad hoc basis by U.S. government grants to research scientists. This lapse in protection of the public health is compounded by the limited and misleading information on pesticide hazards that the general public receives (GAO, 1986b, p. 28).

Clinical scientists are also in the dark about the hazards of most pesticides. For example, the preface to a recent text on the neurotoxicity of pesticides describes a case of exposure to an organophosphate insecticide, and the impetus for writing a book on pesticide toxicity (Ecobichon and Joy, 1982):

". . . . The duration of subtle central and neuromuscular effects of this particular agent was a surprise, 'toxicity' being observed long after the patient was considered to have recovered on the basis of normal values for erythrocytic and plasma cholinesterase analysis. Psychiatric sequelae were observed for at least three months after the so-called 'recovery.' Episodes of fatigue and muscular weakness persisted for several months, becoming less frequent and latterly occurring only after exertion. Continual observation of the patient along with discussions with her physicians were never conclusive but did suggest that something was still amiss. Being intrigued that such effects could occur following exposure to a widely used, seemingly 'safe' insecticide, a search of the literature was begun only to find that, in general, such signs were either unobserved, overlooked, or dismissed as having no relationship to the poisoning. In many cases, once the inhibited enzymatic activities approached normal values, observation of the patients ceased and no extended follow-up of the individual's well being occurred. There was, however, sufficient published literature mentioning long-term physical and behavioral effects to whet the curiosity.

An examination of the literature revealed that such signs and symptoms were not restricted to acute and chronic poisoning by organophosphorous agents but were observed following exposure to chlorinated hydrocarbon insecticides . . ."

Chlordane and heptachlor are chlorinated hydrocarbon insecticides. The CNS is the important locus of action of these compounds. Because mice are much less sensitive to their effects than dogs or humans, studies of cyclodiene toxicity in mice is of limited benefit (Ecobichon and Joy, 1982).

Matsumura and Tanaka (1984) summarized the molecular basis of neurotoxicity actions of cyclodiene-type insecticides. Cyclodienes interact with the picrotoxinin receptor in the nervous system. Cyclodiene poisoning increases the release of excitatory transmitters at the central nervous system. The authors believe that cyclodiene insecticides interfere with the GABA neurotransmission system.

The synapse is the primary target of cyclodiene insecticides. Those synapses characterized as having high numbers of converging pre-synaptic elements whose net activity serves to modulate the excitability of the post-synaptic cells are the most sensitive. At these synapses, the response of the post-synaptic cell to afferent input increases, leading to a lowered threshold of excitation and to an increase in the number and frequency of action potentials generated as a response. This process ''avalanches'' along post-synaptic pathways, ultimately producing responses 10 to 100 times more intense than normal (Ecobichon and Joy, 1982).

This hyperresponsiveness is thought to arise because: (1) inhibitory activity is depressed or blocked, or (2) excitatory input is increased (Ecobichon and Joy, 1982).

The preponderance of the symptoms developing after exposure are the direct result of the CNS action. Early symptoms of acute poisoning include evidence of motor hyperexcitability which may include myoclonic jerking and convulsions. Headache, nausea, vomiting, general malaise, and dizziness may or may not be experienced (Ecobichon and Joy, 1982).

Chronic exposure to cyclodiene insecticides may produce persisting alterations in neurological and psychological functions. Psychological disorders that can result include anxiety, irritability, insomnia, and motor pathology. Children who are poisoned may develop mental retardation and hyperactivity.

Case Reports

Stevens (1970) reported a case of chlordane toxicity in a woman using a mothproofer to spray clothing. Chronic neurologic and psychologic disease ensued. Garrettson et al. (1985) reported a case of subacute chlordane poisoning with various nervous system dysfunctions. Myoclonic jerking occured after a delay of one month. The subject was lost to long-term follow-up.

Singer (1987) presented a case involving chlordane where chronic nervous system function was manifest. A man was exposed to chlordane in a contaminated house for eight months, during which time he underwent personality and other psychological changes. He began having temper tantrums and fistfights, and suffered from claustrophobia, impotence, fatigue, and restlessness. He left employment as a senior draftman. Air sampling of the house found 856 $\mu g/m^3$ heptachlor and 1,097 $\mu g/m^3$ chlordane, 4 times the threshold limit value for U.S. workers. Chlordane was 146 ppb in his blood and 8.8 ppm in his fat, which was considered above "background" levels.

By the time of the examination (seven years post-exposure), symptoms had resolved to some extent. Tests administered included the Wechsler Adult Intelligence Scale (WAIS-R), Benton Visual Retention Test, the Wechsler Memory Scale: Logical Memory, Grooved Pegboard Test, Trailmaking, malingering tests, and conduction tests of the median motor, median sensory and sural nerves, bilaterally. Deficits were found on the Object Assembly Subtest of the WAIS-R and the Memory Scale Tests, indicating functional deficits in visuospatial organization, and recent and delayed auditory memory, with borderline findings on the Visual Retention Test, indicating possible deficits in recent visual memory. Peripheral nerve response was within normal limits. Although the test results were not definitive by themselves, with alternative explanations ruled out, it seemed more probable than not that chlordane toxicity contributed to or caused the emotional disturbance in this man.

Singer and Scott (1987) reported a case of aldrin neurotoxicity. Aldrin is a related cyclodiene pesticide. A 37-year-old female subject was examined after acute domestic environmental exposure to a cyclodiene insecticide. The subject reported suffering from memory dysfunction, headaches, concentration problems, loss of sexual interest, depression, anxiety, mood changes, and sleep disturbance. Neuropsychological testing was conducted 21 months post-exposure.

Premorbid full scale intellectual functioning in the average range had been measured previous to exposure using the Lorge-Thorndike Scale. Post-exposure intellectual functioning was measured using the Wechsler Adult Intelligent Scale-Revised (WAIS-R). Post-exposure full scale intellectual functioning was measured in the low average range, a significant decrement in intellect by 21 points. Other neuropsychological tests were included in the assessment battery. Results indicated impairment in virtually every ability measured, including deficits in short-term memory, logical thinking, visuospatial ability, psychomotor reaction time, recent visual memory, recent and delayed auditory logical memory, figure-ground relationships, manual dexterity, visuomotor tracking, mental flexibility, information processing and tracking, and auditory attention. A diagnosis of cyclodiene insecticide toxicity was supported.

Spyker et al. (1989) reported a study of 68 people who presented with concerns about chlordane home poisonings. They found elevated symptoms of headache, fatigue, memory deficits, personality changes, decreased attention span, numbness or paresthesias, disorientation, and seizures. Electromyography (EMG) was abnormal in 22% of those examined; electronystagmography (ENG) was abnormal in 63%, and neuropsychiatric testing was abnormal in 56%.

Regulatory Actions

The NRC (1982) found that "Given the available data . . . the Committee concluded that it could not determine a level of exposure to any of the [cyclodiene] termiticides below which there would be no biologic effects . . . [E]very effort should be made to minimize exposure to the greatest extent feasible . . .

Because of the shortcomings of current data and in the view of the Committee's request that more definitive data be developed, the airborne concentration of 5 $\mu g/m^2$ should be regarded as an interim guideline for exposure not exceeding 3 years. This 3 year period is suggested with the expectation that it will provide adequate time for the needed health data to begin developing."

In an EPA draft document of August 21, 1986, the EPA found that the misuse and/or misapplication of termiticides often results in significant exposure and potential risk to human health. The reports indicated that chlordane was the most frequently misused or misapplied termiticides (EPA, 1986).

New York state has permanently banned chlordane application. This ban was based on the findings that "the chlorinated cyclodienes have a demonstrated ability to attack sites within the central nervous system. They are toxic to the liver. They persist in the environment, accumulate in humans and animals, and are excreted in the milk of nursing mothers thereby exposing infants to unnecessary health risks. They are difficult, if not impossible to remove from the environment. Their persistence and toxicity has resulted in documented environmental residue and toxicity in New York fish and wildlife. Their use as termiticides has resulted in numerous human exposures with accompanying health risks. The potential for future exposures should be eliminated.

There are effective and acceptable alternatives to chlorinated hydrocarbons and the continued use of cyclodienes offers risks to the general public and the environment that cannot be easily mitigated. For these reasons, the continued use of the chlorinated cyclodienes cannot be justified." (NYS, 1986)

The report listed the five basic methods which may be used for preventing or controlling termite infestations. These are: (1) structural modification; (2) chemical control; (3) use of termite resistant wood; (4) biologic control; and (5) integrated pest management.

The report found that "it is not uncommon for structures treated with chlordane to be reinfested within 10 years of the initial treatment and sometimes retreatment is required as soon as 1 to 2 years after the initial treatment." The report found that contamination of interior air and surfaces occurs where there have been chlordane subterranean applications (NYS, 1986).

Under current agreement with EPA (New York Times, 1987), Velsicol will cease to sell chlordane for consumer use in the United States (although they still have permission to continue to export chlordane) until the company can show that an application method could prevent pesticide residue from seeping into the treated residence. The agreement was prompted by a Velsicol study of 40 homes that had been treated according to label directions with pesticides containing chlordane and heptachlor, all of which showed low but consistent airborne concentrations of the chemicals. By not allowing any amounts of chlordane residue in living areas, EPA implies that any amount of chlordane may pose a human health risk.

Nevertheless, one year later (AP, 1988), the EPA allowed chlordane to be applied at 150 residences around the country. Air will be monitored for 2 years to detect any levels of chlordane. These tests will occur, even though EPA said that detectable levels of chlordane inside houses raised "concerns that long-term exposure to low levels of chlordane could pose health risks, including the increased risk of developing cancer." Chlordane has already been applied to 30 million homes in the U.S.

REFERENCES

AP. 1988. EPA allows home testing of banned termite killer. *Rockland Journal News*, August 7, 1988. p. H10.

Ecobichon, D. and Joy, R. 1982. *Pesticides and Neurological Diseases*. CRC Press; Boca Raton, Florida.

EPA. 1986. Restricted use classification of pesticides used for subterranean termite control and consumer advisory sheet distribution; Criteria and procedures. August 21, 1986.

GAO 1986a. Pesticides: EPA's formidable task to assess and regulate their risks. United States General Accounting Office, GAO/RCED-86-125. Washington, D.C.

GAO 1986b. Nonagricultural pesticides: Risks and regulations. United States General Accounting Office, GAO/RCED-86-89. Washington, D.C.

Garrettson, L. K., Guzelian, P. S., and Blanke, R. V. 1984. Subacute chlordane poisoning, *J. Toxicol.—Clin. Toxicol.* 22(6):565–571.

Gosselin, R. E., Smith, R. P., and Hodge, H. T. 1984. *Clinical Toxicology of Commercial Products*. 5th Ed. Williams and Wilkins: Baltimore.

Matsumura, F. and Tanaka, K. 1984. The molecular basis of neurotoxicity actions of cyclodiene-type insecticides. In *Cellular and Molecular Neurotoxicity*. Raven Press: New York.

National Research Council, Committee on Toxicology. 1979. *Chlordane in Military Housing*. National Academy of Science: Washington, D.C.

National Research Council. 1977. *An Evaluation of the Carcinogenicity of Chlordane and Heptachlor*. National Academy of Science: Washington, D.C.

National Research Council. 1982. *An Assessment of the Health Risks of Seven Pesticides Used for Termite Control*. National Academy Press: Washington, D.C.

New York Times. 1987. Maker to stop sale of 2 cancer-tied pesticides. August 12, 1987. p. A15.

NYS. 1986. Draft environmental impact statement on amendments to 6 NYCRR Part 326 relating to the restriction of the pesticides aldrin, chlordane, chlorpyrofos, dieldrin and heptachlor. 2/86, NYS DEC.

Singer, R. and Scott, N. 1987. Neuropsychological evaluation of cyclodiene insecticide toxicity. *Toxicol.* 7(1):248.

Singer, R. 1987. Forensic evaluation of chlordane neurotoxicity. Paper presented at the First Annual Meeting of the International Neurotoxicity Association.

Spyker, D. A., Bond, R. R., Jylkka, M., and Bernad, P. G. 1989. Subacute home chlordane poisoning: Fact or fallacy. *Vet. Hum. Toxicol.* 31:(4) 356. August 1989.

Stevens, H. Neurotoxicity of some common halogenated hydrocarbons. 1970. In *Laboratory Diagnosis of Diseases Caused by Toxic Agents.* St. Louis, Missouri: Warren H. Green.

FORMALDEHYDE NEUROTOXICITY

Formaldehyde is ubiquitous in the natural and man-made environment. It is critical to the metabolic pathway of the methyl group, one of the body's key units of metabolism (Golberg, 1983).

Biologically Important Reactions. Formaldehyde is a normal metabolite in mammalian systems, and in small quantities, is rapidly metabolized. The adverse effects of formaldehyde may be related to its high reactivity (its affinity to form chemical bonds) with amines, nucleic acids, histones, proteins, and amino acids. It reacts with amino groups in RNA and DNA by breaking down hydrogen bonds. If permanent cross-links are formed between DNA reactive sites and formaldehyde, these links could interfere with replication of DNA and may result in a mutation (Newall, 1983).

Formaldehyde goes into solution when in contact with body tissues. It replaces the active hydrogen in DNA, RNA, and other protein molecules. Alkylation of protein causes tissue fixation or preservation and disinfection (Feinman, 1988).

The study of formaldehyde effects began as early as 1640 when Fischer, a noted chemist of his day, began to investigate a component of insect venom, formic acid. Even before the twentieth century, formaldehyde was used in leather tanning, embalming, tissue preservation, and the manufacture of textiles (Garry et al., 1980).

Use. Formaldehyde gas in solution is found in such household products as antiseptics, deodorizing preparations, and fumigants. It may leach out of housing insulation made from urea formaldehyde foam insulation (UFFI) (Gosselin et al., 1984), and may be present in the home from other synthetic building materials. Formaldehyde resin finishes are used in textile manufacture to create wrinkle resistance and permanent press fabrics. It is also used as the starting material in the production of hard plastics (Feinman, 1988).

American manufacturers produce over 6 billion pounds of formaldehyde a year. Formaldehyde is usually manufactured by reacting methanol vapor and air over a catalyst. It is sold mainly as a water-based solution called formalin, which is 37% to 50% formaldehyde by weight. The widespread use of formaldehyde arises in part because of its high reactivity, colorless nature, purity in commercial form, and low cost. In making other chemicals, it can link similar and dissimilar molecules together.

Formaldehyde is used to produce synthetic resins such as urea-, phenol-, and melanin formaldehyde resins. These resins are used primarily as adhesives when making particleboard, fiberboard, and plywood. The textile industry uses formaldehyde for producing creaseproof, crushproof, flame resistant, and shrinkproof fabrics. The use of formaldehyde in embalming fluids is now required by all state laws (NIOSH, 1981).

Derivatives. Formaldehyde is also known as methanal. It is generally sold commercially as an aqueous solution, formalin, which contains at least 37% formaldehyde. As formalin ages during storage, polymerization or decomposition to formic acid may occur. The solid formaldyhyde polymer, paraformaldehyde, is also available commercially. Trioxane and tetraoxane are additional commercial variations of formaldehyde, used in applications including textile finishing (Feinman, 1988).

Exposure. NIOSH estimated that in the early 1970s, 1.6 million workers were exposed to formaldehyde in more than 60 industries. Formaldehyde in the environment can originate from many sources, including incinerators, photochemical smog, and engine exhaust (NIOSH, 1981).

Indoor sources of air pollution from formaldehyde have been identified both by association with high ambient levels and by direct measurement of emission rates. The strongest sources are articles fabricated with urea-formaldehyde resins that are used in large amounts in the indoor environment. Examples include urea formaldehyde foam insulation (UFFI), plywood, paneling, and particle board underlays or decking. Medium-density fiberboard is a sufficiently strong emitter that even smaller articles such as furniture can elevate indoor levels of formaldehyde significantly (NCTR, 1984).

Most consumers are possibly exposed to formaldehyde gas through its use in construction materials, wood products, textiles, home furnishings, paper, cosmetics, and pharmaceuticals. Two subpopulations at special risk are the 2.2 million residents of mobile homes which contain particle board and plywood, with an average exposure of 0.4 ppm formaldehyde; and the 1.7 million persons living in conventional homes insulated with UFFI, potential average exposure of 0.12 ppm.

Automobiles emit 610 million pounds of formaldehyde each year. The chemical has a short half-life in air, because it is degraded by photochemical processes, and also is unstable in water (NIH, 1985).

Pressed wood products and formaldehyde use, will be discussed later in this section.

General Toxicity of Formaldehyde

Formaldehyde is rated as moderately to very toxic (approximately 1 ounce oral dose will kill the average 150 lb. person; Gosselin et al. 1984). Formaldehyde is detectable by most people at levels below 1 ppm. It produces mild sensory irritation of the eyes, nose, and throat at 2 to 5 ppm, becomes unpleasant at 5 to 10 ppm, and is intolerable at levels in excess of 25 ppm (Clayton and Clayton, 1981). With high concentrations, coughing, dysphagia (difficulty in swallowing), bronchitis, pneumonia, edema or spasm of the larynx can occur (Gosselin et al., 1984). Human deaths have resulted from massive inhalation of formaldehyde (Clayton and Clayton, 1981). Occupational exposures to the gas frequently induces asthma, and allergic type reactions have been reported in some individuals at concentrations below the odor threshold of about 0.8 ppm (Gosselin et al., 1984).

Ingestion can damage the laryngeal, esophageal, and gastric membranes at high doses. Systemic symptoms include nausea, vomiting, hematemesis (vomiting of blood), abdominal pain, hematuria (blood in urine), anuria (total suppression of urine formation), vertigo, fright, convulsions, and stupor. Aspiration of the formaldehyde solutions into the lungs can quickly cause respiratory distress (Gosselin et al., 1984).

Formaldehyde as a gas or in solution will react as a primary irritant on skin, causing an erythematous or eczematous dermatitis reaction on exposed areas. Allergic-type sensitization can result. The widespread use of formaldehyde resins to improve the durability and crease resistance of fabrics has resulted in the exposure of garment workers, sales personnel, and the general public to the resins and to low levels of formaldehyde released from fabrics. Contact dermatitis occasionally results, especially on areas of the body where the garments chafe the wearer or where body heat and evaporation are concentrated, such as the neck and thighs (Clayton and Clayton, 1981).

Following the widespread use of formaldehyde resins in homes in the northeast United States in the 1970s, complaints ranging from eye and throat irritation, to breathing difficulties, headache, nausea, sleeplessness, skin rashes, and epistaxis came to the attention of health agencies (Gosselin et al., 1984).

The U.S. Consumer Product Safety Commission (CPSC) reported that over 5,000 persons complained to them of adverse health effects believed to be associated with UFFI (CPSC, 1982). The symptoms included eye, nose, throat, and skin irritation, breathing difficulties, nausea, vomiting, headaches, dizziness, irritability, insomnia, and sensitization. CPSC conducted an in-depth investigation of 384 cases. The data was analyzed in a number of ways. CPSC concluded that the problem of UFFI toxicity was real, and banned the product in residential and school buildings in 1982. The ban was later vacated by the U.S. Court of Appeals (NIH, 1985).

The principle noticeable effect of low concentrations of formaldehyde in humans is irritation of the eyes and mucous membranes (NRC, 1981). Table 6-1 shows the reported health effects of formaldehyde at various concentrations.

Carcinogenicity. Formaldehyde vapor is carcinogenic in rats; squamous cell carcinomas of the nasal cavity have been reported (Gosselin et al., 1984).

Excessively high rates of brain cancer and leukemia were found among embalmers, anatomists and pathologists. In further studies of industrial workers, these effects were less common, although increased cancer of the nose and throat were found (Marcus and Feinman, 1988).

The U.S. Consumer Product Safety Commission, in cooperation with the Interagency Regulatory Liaison Group, convened a panel of scientists from eight different federal agencies under the auspices of the National Toxicology Program, and stated, "It is the conclusion of the Panel that it is prudent to regard formaldehyde as posing a carcinogenic risk to humans" (NIOSH, 1981). In 1987, the EPA continued to classify formaldehyde as a "probable human carcinogen" (EPA, 1987).

Summary of the Major Systemic Responses to Formaldehyde. Skin irritation occurs in some people when they are exposed to a less than 1% solution of formaldehyde. Clinically relevant allergic hypersensitivity reactions to 2% formaldehyde were observed in 4% of dermatitis patients. Nose, throat, and upper respiratory tract irritation are common effects of formaldehyde inhalation. Typ-

Table 6-1. Reported health effects of formaldehyde at various concentrations (Adapted from NRC, 1981).

Health Effects Reported	Approximate Formaldehyde Concentration, ppm
Neurophysiologic effects	0.05–1.50
Odor threshold	0.05–1.0
Eye irritation	0.01–2.0*
Upper airway irritation	0.10–25
Lower airway and pulmonary effects	5–30
Pulmonary edemas, inflammation, pneumonia	50–100
Death	100+

*The low concentration (0.01 ppm) was observed in the presence of other pollutants that may have been acting synergistically.

ical symptoms include coughing, tightness of the nose and chest, and wheezing. Asthma may occur. Structural and functional changes of the CNS, peripheral nerves, and sensory organs have been found after formaldehyde exposure. The production of pain by formaldehyde is used as a standard pharmacological test system in animals. Formaldehyde can cause delayed-type hpersensitivity, and allergic contact dermatitis, a manifestation of delayed-type hypersensitivity. A variety of other immunologic effects have also been noted (Feinman, 1988).

Consensus Decisions and Regulatory Action

The National Research Council found that there was no population threshold for the irritant effects of formaldehyde. Even at extremely low airborne concentrations, a proportion of the population will respond with irritation. The Committee recommended that formaldehyde be kept at the lowest practical concentrations in indoor residential air (NRC, 1981).

As of 1981, the OSHA standard for formaldehyde was 3 ppm, as a time-weighted average over 8 hours. NIOSH has recommended a workplace ceiling limit of 1 ppm (NRC, 1981). In 1987, OSHA set the level at which protective action is required at 0.5 ppm. This standard was recently upheld by a federal appeals court, although certain questions of the standard are still being litigated (AP, 1989).

In the U.S. there is no standard for formaldehyde for 24-hour-continuous, non-occupational exposure, as occurs in residences. The American Hygiene Association recommended an outdoor, airborne standard of .1 ppm. The National Research Council has stated that airborne formaldehyde in manned spacecrafts should not exceed .1 ppm. Northern European countries have residential standards of .1 ppm. The American Society of Heating, Refrigeration, and Air-Conditioning Engineers set a comfort ceiling of .1 ppm (NRC, 1981).

Neurotoxicity of Formaldehyde

Animal Biochemical Neurotoxicity Studies. In a study of the pathways of formaldehyde biochemistry, radioactivity was found in the brain from blood circulation after animals were exposed to the radioactive marker 14 C-formaldehyde after 6 hours of exposure (NCTR, 1984).

Neurochemical Studies. In humans, formaldehyde is mainly metabolized to formate, an inhibitor of cytochrome oxidase. Because of the evolutionary loss of the enzymes uricase and formyltetrahydrofolate reductase, human beings cannot metabolize formate in many syntheses via the folate pathway. This enhances the human toxicity of chemicals that are metabolized to formate. The actual neurochemical cause of neurotoxicity is hypothesized to be hypoxia and acidosis (NCTR, 1984; Gosselin et al., 1984).

Morphologic Changes in Response to Formaldehyde Exposure. Bonashevskaya (1973) reported lesions in the central amygdaloid complex of rats after three months exposure to 1 to 3 mg/m^3 formaldehyde (NCTR, 1984). In another study, a three month exposure to formaldehyde concentration of 1 mg/m^3 produced changes in brain structure and neuromuscular function. Proliferation of glial cells was evident and synaptic structures were not well formed (Feldman and Bonashevskaya, 1971).

Human Neurotoxicity Studies

Experimental Sensitivity Studies. Odor threshold for formaldehyde was 0.06 ppm for 7 of 15 subjects (Feldman and Bonashevskaya, 1971). Evaluating the EEG in 5 of the subjects most sensitive to formaldehyde exposure, they reported that concentrations below the odor threshold of .04 ppm produced changes in EEG.

Epidemiologic Studies of Symptoms. The results of such studies are controversial and beyond the scope of this paper. See NCTR, 1984, for a summary of these studies.

Occupational Exposure. Workers exposed to formaldehyde have reported symptoms which are suggestive of nervous system involvement, including headaches, weakness, dizziness, sensory disturbances, irritability, tremors of the limbs, irregular respiration, and fluctuations of body temperature (Ahmad and Whitson, 1973; Miller, 1979; NIH, 1945; found in Sauter, 1981). Headache, dizziness and nausea, indicative of CNS effects, have been reported by others (Arbeta & Halsa, 1978).

Other investigators of occupational formaldehyde exposure found excitation, insomnia, anorexia, tremor, weakness, vision disorders, paresthesias, pain, and temperature hypersensitivity (Lazerev and Levina, 1976; found in Anger and Johnson, 1985).

Case Reports. Occasional case reports describing nervous system effects of formaldehyde have appeared, including descriptions of "acute nervous manifestations," mental confusion, memory deficits, poor concentration and depression (Sauter, 1981).

Some case report data concerning the behavioral effects of formaldehyde in children is available. Behavioral disturbances, including fatigue, restlessness, irritability, and attention problems were reported in pre-school children after the children moved to a mobile home where there were noticeable formaldehyde fumes (Sauter, 1981).

Sauter (1981) reported a case of an 8 year old boy, exposed for 2 years to formaldehyde vapors. During this period, WISC IQ dropped from the 91st to the 70th percentile, with the greatest decrease in performance measures. A decrease from the 70th to the 12th percentile was found on the memory scale of the McCarthy Scales of Children's Abilities. School personnel reported symptoms of lethargy, attention deficits, and other problems. Westgate (1980; found in Sauter, 1981) reported exposure-related seizures in 3 children.

While these case reports are not complete, they suggest the possibility of neurobehavioral deterioration from formaldehyde exposure.

Experimental Studies. Sauter (1981) compared 32 formaldehyde exposed children with unexposed controls. When socioeconomic status was statistically removed as a variable, only the memory tasks of the battery of tests differentiated the groups. Higher activity levels and left-handedness was associated with prenatal exposure.

Bach et al. (1987) exposed 61 subjects for 5.5 hours to controlled amounts of formaldehyde in a climate chamber (0.0; 0.15; 0.40 and 1.20 mg/m³). Subjects with 5 years occupational exposure to formaldehyde ($N = 32$) were matched with 29 subjects on the basis of gender, age, education, and smoking habits. On the basis of psychometric testing prior to experimental exposure, formaldehyde workers had the lowest scores and the most errors. The results were mixed when acute exposures were tested. The results suggested that CNS functions as measured by short-term memory, attention, and ability to concentrate are decreased by formaldehyde exposure, but the authors recommended further studies to verify the effect.

Schenker et al. (1982) studied 24 residents of 6 homes which contained UFFI. Thirty-nine percent reported problems with headaches, memory, concentration, and emotional stability. Fourteen of the 18 adults were tested with a limited battery of neuropsychological tests. Of the 6 with memory complaints, 4 showed abnormal Digit Span Test results. Eleven of the 14 who were tested had impairment in either their attention span or their capacity to sustain attention. Depression was found in 9 subjects. The authors concluded that "chronic low-level exposure to formaldehyde may cause significant mental status changes. However, the sample size in this pilot study was small and may have been biased by self-referrals."

Kilburn et al. (1987) tested 305 histology technicians and analyzed the data using regression analysis. Histology technicians are exposed to formaldehyde, toluene, and xylene, and have been found to have an increased prevalence of disturbances of memory, mood, equilibrium, sleep, and to suffer from headaches and indigestion.

The subjects were tested with an hour-long battery of neuropsychological tests designed to evaluate the previously listed symptoms. The subjects had worked an average of 17 years as histology technicians. Self-reported exposure to formaldehyde fumes, based on detection of odor, averaged 4.3 hours per day.

After controlling for age effects, increased daily hours of exposure to formaldehyde were correlated with reduced performance on 3 of 8 memory tests (including logical memory, visual memory, and digit span), errors on Trails A, pegboard, and Sharpened-Romberg. Estimated exposure to solvents was only associated with diminished recall of stories.

Based upon current laboratory measurements, the authors estimated that formaldehyde concentrations were about 1 ppm, with peaks of 5 ppm. Because histological methods have changed very little in 40 years, these measurements were thought to approximate the levels of formaldehyde over the years of exposure.

Kilburn et al. (1985a) studied the neurobehavioral effects of occupational formaldehyde exposure in four groups of workers ($N = 89$), including fiberglass workers whose formaldehyde exposure occurred as part of the fiberglass manufacturing process. They found that the frequency of neurobehavioral symptoms, such as problems with sleep, memory, and mood, increased with increasing levels of formaldehyde exposure. The authors concluded that although there were a broad range of other types of exposures, the results were sufficiently clear to show the effects of formaldehyde neurotoxicity.

Kilburn et al. (1985b; 1983) also studied 76 histotechnologists who were exposed to formaldehyde, and found that increasing levels of formaldehyde exposure correlated with neurobehavioral symptoms such as disturbances of memory, mood, equilibrium, and sleep. The correlation of formaldehyde exposure with neurobehavioral symptoms was stronger than the correlation of such symptoms and exposure to xylene and toluene.

Cripe and Dodrill (1988) studied 13 subjects "involved in personal injury litigation alleging brain dysfunction due to chronic exposure to formaldehyde." At the time of testing, the subjects had been removed from the exposure for a mean of 21 months. They had been exposed to formaldehyde for an average of 37 months ($SD = 12$), at a mean exposure level of .31 ppm ($SD = .15$). No further description of exposure levels, patterns of exposure, daily duration of exposure (if daily), source of exposure, or whether the subjects were exposed in the same or multiple exposure settings was provided. They were compared with a group of mild head injured patients, and a group of controls drawn from the community. The variables controlled were sex, age, and years of education. The mild head injured group had subtle to mild neurobehavioral dysfunction.

The formaldehyde and control group performed similarly, and both differed from the mild head injured group. The formaldehyde and mild brain injured group were similar for MMPI findings, compared with the control group.

The authors suggested caution in drawing conclusions of brain damage in persons with chronic low-level formaldehyde exposure. The authors further offered some cautions when generalizing from their data: further research is needed with larger samples and controls; study of the acute neuropsychological effects of formaldehyde is needed; and further research is needed with an expanded battery of neuropsychological tests that may be more appropriate for evaluating the behavioral toxicology of attention, memory, and subtle impairment.

Sufficient evidence exists to consider the possibility of brain dysfunction from formaldehyde exposure. A person whose cognition, emotions, and behavior have deteriorated following formaldehyde exposure should have a complete and sensitive neuropsychological examination, along with nerve conduction velocity assessment. Workers with continued exposure to formaldehyde should be monitored for early signs of neurotoxicity.

REFERENCES

Ahmad, I. and Whitson, T. C. 1973. Formaldehyde: How much of a hazard? *Industrial Medicine and Surgery* 42(8):26–27.

Anger, W. and Johnson, B. 1985. Chemicals affecting behavior. In J. O'Donoghue, Ed. *Neurotoxicity of Industrial and Commercial Chemicals.* Vol. 1. CRC Press: Boca Raton, Florida.

AP. 1989. Review of limit on gas is ordered. *The New York Times.* June 10, 1989.

Arbeta and Halsa. 1987. Scandinavian expert TLV's, Formaldehyde (in Swedish). Found in Bach, B., Molhave, L., and Pedersen, O. F. Human reactions during controlled exposures to low concentrations of formaldehyde—performance tests. *Proceedings of the 4th International Conference on Indoor Air Quality and Climates.* West Berlin. 17–21 August 1987. Volume 2, Institute for Water, Soil and Air Hygiene.

Bach, B., Molhave, L., and Pedersen, O. F. 1987. Human reactions during controlled exposures to low concentrations of formaldehyde—performance tests. *Proceedings of the 4th International Conference on Indoor Air Quality and Climates.* West Berlin. 17–21 August 1987. Volume 2, Institute for Water, Soil and Air Hygiene.

Bonashevskaya, T. I. 1973. Amygdaloid lesions after exposure to formaldehyde. *Arkh. Anat. Gistol.-Embriol.* 6:56–59.

Clayton, G. D. and Clayton, F. E. 1981. *Patty's Industrial Hygiene and Toxicology.* John Wiley & Sons: New York. pp. 2629–2669.

CPSC. 1984a. *United States Consumer Product Safety Commission: Questions and Answers on Pressed Wood Products.* U.S. Printing Office.

CPSC. 1984b. *United States Consumer Product Safety Commission: Status Report on Formaldehyde Emissions from Pressed Wood Products.* U.S. Printing Office.

CPSC. 1982. Consumer Product Safety Commission. Ban of urea-formaldehyde foam insulation. *Fed. Register* 47(64):14366–14419, April 2, 1982.

Cripe, L. I. and Dodrill, C. B. 1988. Neuropsychological test performances with chronic low-level formaldehyde exposure. *Clinical Neuropsychologist,* 2(1):41–48.

EPA. 1987. *US EPA Office of Toxic Substances: Fact Sheet on Formaldehyde.* April 16, 1987.

Feinman, Susan E. 1988. *Formaldehyde Sensitivity and Toxicity.* CRC Press: Boca Raton, Florida.

Feldman, Y. G. and Bonashevskaya, T. I. 1971. On the effects of low concentrations of formaldehyde. *Hygiene and Sanitation,* 36(5):174–180.

Garry, V. F., Oatman, L. O., Pleus, R., and Gray, D. 1980. *Formaldehyde in the*

Home: Some Environmental Disease Perspectives. Minnesota Department of Health, February, 1980.

Golberg, L. 1983. Forward. In *Formaldehyde Toxicity* (J. E. Gibson, Ed.), Hemisphere Publishing Co.: Washington, D.C.

Gosselin, R. E., Smith, R. P., and Hodge, H. C. 1984. Clinical Toxicology of Commercial Products. Williams & Wilkins: Baltimore. Section III, pp. 196–198.

Kilburn, K. H., Warshaw, R., and Thornton, J. C. 1987. Formaldehyde impairs memory, equilibrium and dexterity in histology technicians: Effects which persist for days after exposure. *Arch. Env. Health* 42(2):117–120.

Kilburn, K. H. et al. 1985a. Pulmonary and neurobehavioral effects of formaldehyde exposure. *Arch. Env. Health* 40(5):254–260.

Kilburn, K. H. et al. 1985b. Neurobehavioral and respiratory symptoms of formaldehyde and xylene exposure in histology technicians. *Arch. Env. Health* 40(4):229–233.

Kilburn, K. H. et al. 1983. Toxic effects of formaldehyde and solvents in histology technicians: A preliminary report. *J. Histotechnology* 6(2):73–76.

Lazerev, N. V. and Levina, E. N. 1976. *Harmful Substances in Industry.* Khimiya Press: Leningrad. (Transl. by Literature Research, Annandale, VA.)

Marcus, S. C. and Feinman, S. E. 1988. Formaldehyde and cancer epidemiology. In Feinman, Susan E. *Formaldehyde Sensitivity and Toxicity.* 1988. CRC Press: Boca Raton, Florida.

Miller, C. S. 1979. Mass psychogenic illness or chemically induced hypersusceptibility. Paper prepared for *Symposium on the Diagnosis and Amelioration of Mass Psychogenic Illness.* U.S. Department of Health, Education, and Welfare; Center for Disease Control.

NAS. 1980. *Formaldehyde—An Assessment of Its Health Effects.* Report to the Consumer Product Safety Commission. National Academy of Science: Washington, D.C.

Newall, G. W. 1983. Overview of formaldehyde. In *Formaldehyde Toxicity* (J. E. Gibson, Ed.), Hemisphere Publishing Co.: Washington, D.C.

NIH. 1945. *Formaldehyde: Its Toxicity and Potential Danger* (Supplement No. 181 to the Public Health Reports). Washington, D.C., U.S. Government Printing Office.

NIH. 1985. *Fourth Annual Report on Carcinogens.* National Technical Information Service, PB85-134633.

NCTR. 1984. *Report on the Consensus Workshop on Formaldehyde.* Environmental Health Perspectives, Vol. 58, pp. 328–321. DHHS Publication No. (NIH) 84-218.

NIOSH. 1981. *Formaldehyde: Evidence of Carcinogenicity.* Current Intelligence Bulletin 34. April 15, 1981.

NRC. 1981. *Formaldehydes and Other Aldehydes.* National Academy Press: Washington, D.C.

O'Donoghue, J. L. (Ed.). 1985. *Neurotoxicity of Industrial and Commercial Chemicals.* Volume I, CRC Press, Boca Raton, Florida, p. 101.

Sauter, D. L. 1981. *The Development and Application of a Battery for the Exploratory Screening for Neuropsychological Deficits in Children Exposed to Formaldehyde.* (Ph.D. Thesis) University of Wisconsin, Madison.

Schenker, M. B., Weiss, S. T., and Murawski, B. J. 1982. Health effects of residence in homes with urea formaldehyde foam insulation: A pilot study. *Environment International* 8:359–363.

Skiest, (Ed.) 1977. *Handbook of Adhesives*, 2nd Ed., Van Nostrand Reinhold: New York.

Sterling, 1980. *The Encyclopedia of Wood: Wood as an Engineering Material.* Sterling Publishing Co.: New York.

Westgate, H. 1980. *Testimony at the Urea-Formaldehyde Foam Insulation Public Hearing.* Minneapolis, MN. Consumer Product Safety Commission, February 5, 1980.

APPENDIX
PRESSED WOOD PRODUCTS

Plywood.   Plywood is a glued wood panel made up of relatively thin layers, or plies, with the grain of adjacent layers at an angle, usually of 90°. The usual constructions have an odd number of plies. The outside plies are called faces, or face and back plies, the inner plies are called cores or centers, and the plies immediately below the face and back are called crossbands. The core may be veneer, lumber, or particleboard, with the total panel thickness typically not less than 1/16 inch or more than 3 inches. Broadly speaking, two classes of plywood are available—hardwood and softwood. In general, softwood plywood is intended for construction use (sheathing for walls, roofs and floors), and hardwood plywood for uses where appearance is important (Sterling, 1980). Softwood plywood, which is used for exterior applications and flooring in home construction, is manufactured with phenol formaldehyde resins rather than urea formaldehyde (CPSC, 1984a).

Particleboard.   Particleboards are manufactured from small pieces of wood that are glued together with a thermosetting resin or an equivalent binder. Wax sizing is added to all commercially produced particleboards to improve water resistance. Other additions may be introduced during manufacture to improve some property or provide added resistance to fire, decay, or to insects such as termites.

Particleboard is among the newest of the wood-base panel materials. The thermosetting resins used are primarily urea formaldehyde and phenol formaldehyde. Urea formaldehyde is low in cost and is the binder most often used for particleboards intended for interior or other nonsevere exposures. Where moderate water or heat resistance is required, melamine-urea formaldehyde resin blends are used.

The kinds of wood particles used in the manufacture of particleboards range from specifically cut flakes, an inch or more in length and only a few hundredths of an inch thick, to fine particles which approach the size of grains of flour. The synthetic resin solids are usually between 5% and 10% by weight of the dry wood finish. These resins are set by heat as the wood particle-resin blend is compressed (Sterling, 1980). Particleboard is used primarily in kitchen cabinets, shelving, countertops, and floor underlayment (CPSC, 1984a).

Fiberboard.   Fiberboards are made essentially of fiberlike components of wood that are interfelted together in the reconstruction and are characterized by a bond produced by the interfelting. Such boards are frequently classified as fibrous-felted board products. At certain densities, under controlled conditions of hot pressing, rebonding of the lignin affects a further bond in the panel product. Binding agents and other materials may be added during manufacture to increase strength, resistance to fire, moisture, decay, etc. Among the materials added are natural and synthetic resins, preservative chemicals, and drying oils. The woodbase fiber panel materials (building fiberboards) are divided into two groups—insulation board (lower density products), and hardboard (medium to high density products) (Sterling, 1980). Medium density fiberboard is used in furniture, door jambs, shelving, and several other applications (CPSC, 1984a).

Adhesives. Urea formaldehyde resin adhesives are used in the manufacture of building materials such as hardboard plywood and particleboard. Urea resin adhesives are products of the condensation reaction of urea and formaldehyde. Mechanical spreaders are used to apply adhesive to veneer in plywood manufacture (Skiest, 1977).

Melamine formaldehyde resin adhesives were introduced commercially in the United States in the 1930s. Melamine formaldehyde and melamine-urea formaldehyde resin adhesives are colorless in the cured state, so they are used primarily in architectural timbers and hardwood plywood where inconspicuous bondlines are an important factor. Melamine resin adhesives are made by condensation reaction of melamine with formaldehyde. Melamine formaldehyde and urea formaldehyde are compatible, and blends of the two are commonly used as bonding agents in hardwood plywood (Skiest, 1977).

Phenol formaldehyde resins are used primarily in the manufacture of softwood plywood. They are also used as binders for particleboards where a higher degree of durability is required than can be provided by urea binders. In the manufacture of plywood, the phenolic resin adhesive is applied to the wood veneers, usually by roller coating (Skiest, 1977).

Resorcinol formaldehyde or resorcinolic adhesives are condensation products of resorcinol with formaldehyde or with various phenol formaldehyde resoles. They are used in the manufacture of plywood, when fast-curing, durable qualities are paramount (Skiest, 1977).

Formaldehyde Emissions. Concern by consumers for formaldehyde emissions from pressed wood products (particleboard, fiberboard, and plywood) arose because of complaints from mobile home residents. Concern has extended to new conventional homes because of recent changes in construction practices and efforts to make homes more energy efficient. Energy efficiency is achieved by reducing fresh air infiltration, using various types of vapor barriers, for example specially formulated paints, natural and synthetic asphalt and rubber coatings, etc. Reduced air infiltration coupled with increasing use of pressed wood products may cause an increase in the indoor concentrations of formaldehyde, as well as other pollutants (CPSC, 1984b).

As of February 1984, the Consumer Product Safety Commission received 2,700 complaints (involving approximately 5,000 persons) that reported adverse health effects believed to be associated with formaldehyde from pressed wood products (CPSC, 1984b).

The formaldehyde gas released from these wood products is believed to be caused by the use of excess formaldehyde in the resin, and the chemical breakdown of the resin, generating formaldehyde gas (CPSC, 1984a). Aging, decay, and shrinkage of the wood components or the adhesive binder, or both, could conceivably add to the formaldehyde gas emissions.

New homes are generally constructed of wood and wood products. Other building materials such as brick and stone are not as cost effective as wood, and therefore not as widely used. New homes have wooden beams, columns, boards, planks, studs, joists, panels, and shelves, some of which are composed of pressed wood. Formaldehyde is an essential component in the adhesive formulations used in these pressed wood products. These wood products (plywood, particleboard, and fiberboard) could in turn, serve as source areas of formaldehyde gas emissions into the household atmosphere.

Storage areas constructed of pressed wood (shelves, walls, etc.), which are normally kept closed, like cupboards and closets, could act as repositories for formaldehyde gas. Lack of ventilation and circulation would cause any formaldehyde fumes which have been generated to remain and concentrate.

GASOLINE TOXICITY

The toxicology of gasoline is complex. While gasoline per se is moderately toxic (Gosselin et al., 1984), gasoline contains many functional additives, such as antiknock fluids, antioxidants, metal deactivators, corrosion inhibitors, anti-icing agents, pre-ignition preventors, upper cylinder lubricants, dyes, and decolorizers (Sandmeyer, 1981). As these substances remain unspecified, their toxicity can be only guessed. As a general rule, the more reactive a substance is, the more toxic to humans it may be.

In order to increase octane, substances added to gasoline include organic lead, organic manganese, and the BTX group (benzene, toluene, and xylene). All of these substances are neurotoxic. (See earlier in this chapter.)

Organophosphates have also been added to gasoline (Soderman, 1972). These substances may be highly neurotoxic, as are organophosphate pesticides.

Gasoline is a complex mixture of over 200 hydrocarbons. Ingestion of little more than an ounce of gasoline can kill the average person. In children, death has occurred from accidental ingestion of 10 to 15 grams of gasoline (a gram is 1/28 ounce). In adults, ingestion of 20 to 50 grams of gasoline may produce severe symptoms of poisoning. Symptoms of severe gasoline intoxication include loss of consciousness, convulsions, cyanosis, congestion, and capillary hemorrhaging of the lungs and internal organs, followed by death due to circulatory failure; in milder cases, symptoms may include vomiting, vertigo, confusion, and fever (Gosselin et al., 1984).

Gasoline is a skin irritant and a possible allergen. Repeated or chronic dermal contact can cause dried skin, lesions, and other dermatologic conditions. Acute inhalation can cause intense burning of the throat and respiratory system, which can develop into bronchopneumonia. At extremely high concentrations, when oxygen displacement is a factor, asphyxiation can occur. Severe intoxication is accompanied by central nervous system (CNS) effects, coma, and convulsions with epileptiform seizures (Clayton and Clayton, 1981).

Chronic ingestion of approximately 1.8 mg/L has been found to cause vomiting, diarrhea, insomnia, headache, dizziness, anemia, and muscle and neurological symptoms (Clayton and Clayton, 1981).

A study of automobile mechanics and gasoline service station workers in New Hampshire between the years 1975 and 1985 found increased mortality for leukemia, and an increase in mental and psychoneurotic personality disorders. These circumstances were attributed primarily to gasoline exposure (Schwartz, 1987). The study listed potential exposures in the service station industry from gasoline vapors, benzene, solvents, lubricating oils and greases, asbestos (from brake and clutch repair), fiberglass, epoxies, and adhesives, as well as welding fumes, and car and truck exhaust. In analyzing the causes of death of workers in the gasoline service station industry, the study uncovered statistically significant proportionate mortality ratio elevations. The observed number of deaths from mental and psychoneurotic disorders for gasoline service station industry workers was nearly four times the expected number of deaths. The study stated that:

> The patterns of mortality of automobile mechanics and workers in the gasoline service station industry suggest that these tradesmen experience an increased leukemia risk . . . . [A]mong the potentially responsible chemical agents known to be present in service stations and garages, most suspect would be gasoline and other solvents containing benzene . . . . Further, the finding of an excess proportion of deaths from suicide in both groups is consistent with the known neurotoxic potential of solvent exposure . . . . Long-term exposure to solvents can result in memory impairment and behavioral changes, including irritability, depressive symptoms, and emotional instability . . . . In view of the likelihood that work in service stations involves chronic exposure, it is not surprising that auto mechanics and service station workers experience a greater proportion of deaths from suicide.

In finding statistically significant increased incidence of mortality associated with exposure to the neurotoxic and carcinogenic compounds listed above, the study concluded that:

> This analysis suggests that one or more of the exposures experienced by automobile mechanics and service station workers poses a carcinogenic risk. Although numerous agents are suspect, the finding of leukemia excess among automobile mechanics and workers in the gasoline service station industry is consistent with exposure to benzene, a known component of gasoline.

The toxicity of selected components of gasoline, such as benzene, toluene, and xylene, rounds out the picture of gasoline toxicity. These substances are reviewed earlier in this chapter. The following gasoline additives will be reviewed below: organic lead, cadmium, and manganese.

ORGANIC LEAD

General Toxicity of Lead

Symptoms of chronic lead poisoning include gastrointestinal disturbances, anemia, insomnia, weight loss, motor weakness, muscle paralysis, joint pain, and kidney disease (Baselt, 1988). Organic lead is more toxic to the central nervous system than inorganic lead.

The central nervous system effects of lead (damage to the brain and nerves) are the most significant effects in terms of human health and performance. Lead affects the blood in many ways. It causes anemia by shortening the life span of the red blood cells and impairing heme synthesis. (Anemia is uncommon with blood lead levels below 80 μg/dl). Lead also damages the kidneys, leading to gout (pain in the joints, chronic progressive arthritis) (Goyer, 1986).

Although lead poisoning can express itself in many ways, three major clinical syndromes have been described. The alimentary type is characterized by weight loss, constipation and severe abdominal cramps caused by intestinal spasms. The neuromuscular type is characterized by weakness, paralysis, muscle wasting, and painful joints and muscles. This has been called saturnine athralgia or gout. The cerebral type will be described below. Other symptoms of lead poisoning include hypertension, hepatitis, and liver failure. Acute poisoning by ingestion alone sometimes causes diarrhea and less often constipation (Gosselin et al., 1984).

The Neurotoxicity of Lead

At what level is lead neurotoxic? No safe level of lead exposure has been determined. Typical levels of lead in the blood of the general population has been found to be 20 μg/dl blood lead, while 40 to 60 μg/dl blood lead levels have been associated with overt toxicity. Considering individual variation in response, concomitant environmental exposure to other toxic agents, and other predisposing factors of lead toxicity, an alleged margin of safety (comparing 20 μg/dl with 40 μg/dl) seems to disappear. In animal studies, blood lead of 20 to 35 μg/dl was shown to cause neurological deficits (Bondy, 1989). Practically speaking, there probably is no threshold of effect for the neurotoxicity of lead.

The Neurotoxicity of Organic Lead

Exposure to organic lead can cause symptoms of central nervous system toxicity that include insomnia, anxiety, lassitude, tremor, hallucinations, psychotic behavior, and convulsions. Chronic exposure can cause symptoms of inorganic lead poisoning and symptoms of organic lead intoxication of the central nervous system (Baselt, 1988).

Compared with inorganic lead, organic lead is more rapidly absorbed through the skin and lungs. Because it is lipophilic, organic lead has a marked affinity for and an ability to pass into nerve and brain tissue which is very fatty. Organic lead compounds also are relatively long-lived in nervous system tissue (Bondy, 1989).

Although organic lead compounds constitute only a small proportion of the total lead exposure of the general population, organic lead compounds comprise about 20% of the lead found in the brains of the general urban population. This demonstrates that organic lead has a particular affinity for brain tissue and that organic lead has significant neurotoxic potential (Bondy, 1989).

Both organic and inorganic lead can cause neurotoxicity, but organic lead is much more toxic. The increased toxicity of organic lead is due in part to it's ability to more easily penetrate the blood-brain barrier. Both types of lead compete with other metals for space in brain tissue. Both types of lead also have a tendency to destroy certain brain regions, notably the hippocampus, which seems to function as a controller of neuronal hyperactivity and consequent behavioral hyperactivity. Endocrine dysfunction can be seen after exposure to both types of lead. The dysfunctions include reduced testoterone levels. Several hormones and hypothalamic peptides are affected by both types of lead (Bondy, 1989).

The main difference between the toxicity of organic and inorganic lead is the heightened capacity of organic lead compounds to interfere with normal brain chemistry and function (Bondy, 1989).

CADMIUM

Cadmium is a trace contaminant of crude oil. The concentration of cadmium in gasoline has been reported as 10 to 50 $\mu g/l$. Cadmium levels of 20 to 900 $\mu g/l$ have been reported as a gasoline additive (API, 1985a).

General Toxicity of Cadmium

Cadmium is absorbed from the lungs and GI tract. Poisoning by acute inhalation is accompanied by slight discomfort at the time of exposure, followed in 4 to 10 hours by coughing, difficulty in breathing, nausea, pain and tightness in the chest, and a burning sensation. Chronic poisoning damages the kidney (the classical toxicologic response to cadmium is kidney damage) and the nervous system (Babitch, 1988).

Neurotoxicity of Cadmium

Anorexia, anosmia, convulsions, dizziness, headache, insomnia, weakness, and weight loss are associated with cadmium poisoning. Not all of these symptoms are observed in all exposed people. Elevated cadmium levels has been associated with decreased in IQ, associative learning, and memory (Babitch, 1988).

MANGANESE

Methyl cyclopentadienyl manganese tricarbonyl (MMT) has been added to gasoline since at least 1975 (Seth and Chandra, 1988).

General Toxicity of Manganese

". . . Typical metal fume fever may develop after acute exposure to manganese oxide fumes with symptoms of fever, muscle pain, chills and dryness of the mouth and throat. However, chronic overexposure to manganese is more frequently encountered in occupational medicine. This may require a year or more of exposure prior to manifestations of CNS symptoms such as headache, restlessness, irritability, personality changes, hallucinations and hearing impairment. Severe toxicity results in muscle weakness and rigidity, tremor and other extrapyramidal symptoms" (Baselt, 1988).

Neurotoxicity of Manganese

Manganese is classified as a neurotoxicant causing localized CNS lesions. It can cause neuronal degeneration of the brain, specifically at the globus pallidus, caudate nucleus, putamen, and cerebellum. The functional disability resembles the extrapyramidal signs and symptoms of Parkinsonism (Norton, 1986).

Chronic manganese poisoning produces a psychological disorder with symptoms such as irritability, difficulty in walking, speech disturbances, compulsive behavior, a mask-like face and Parkinson-like symptoms (Goyer, 1986).

Some neurological signs and symptoms of manganese poisoning are as follows (Seth and Chandra, 1988):

State of Poisoning	Significant Neurological Disorders
1. Prodromal phase	Apathy, asthenia, anorexia, insomnia, muscular pains, mental excitement, hallucinations, unaccountable laughter, impaired memory, compulsive action, sexual excitement followed by impotence

State of Poisoning	Significant Neurological Disorders
2. Intermediate phase	Speech disturbance, clumsiness of movements, abnormal gait, altered balance, exaggerated reflexes in lower limbs, expressionless face, adiodokinesis, and fine tremors
3. Established phase	Muscular rigidity in both the extremities, staggering gait ("cock walk"), fine tremors, spasmodic laughter, excessive sweating

REFERENCES

API. 1985a. *Cadmium: Environmental and Community Health Impact.* American Petroleum Institute Publication 137C. Washington, D.C. January 1985.

API. 1985b. *Cleaning Petroleum Storage Tanks.* American Petroleum Institute Publication 2015. 3rd Ed. Washington, D.C. September 1985.

Babitch, J. 1988. Cadmium neurotoxicity. In *Metal Neurotoxicity.* Stephen Bondy, Ed. CRC Press: Boca Raton, Florida.

Baselt, R. 1988. *Biological Monitoring Methods for Industrial Chemicals.* Second Edition. PSG Publishing Company: Littleton, Massachusetts.

Bondy, S. 1988. *Metal Neurotoxicity.* CRC Press: Boca Raton, Florida.

Clayton, G. D. and Clayton, F. E. 1981. *Patty's Industrial Hygiene and Toxicology.* New York: John Wiley & Sons. pp. 3291–3300.

Gosselin, R. E., Smith, R. P., and Hodge, H. C. 1984. *Clinical Toxicology of Commercial Products* (5th ed.), Section III., pp. 397–404. Williams and Wilkins: Baltimore, Maryland.

Goyer, R. A. 1986. Toxic effect of metals. In *Casarett and Doull's Toxicology: The Basic Science of Poisons.* Macmillan Publishing Company: New York.

Lauwerys, R. 1982. *Industrial Chemical Exposure: Guidelines for Biological Monitoring.* Biomedical Publications: Davis, California.

Norton, S. 1986. Toxic responses of the central nervous system. In *Casarett and Doull's Toxicology: The Basic Science of Poisons.* Macmillan Publishing Company: New York.

Rho, Y.-M. 1986. Acute stagnent air syndrome. *Amer. J. of Forensic Medicine and Pathology* 7:46–48.

Seth, P. and Chandra, S. 1988. Neurotoxic effects of manganese. In *Metal Neurotoxicity.* Stephen Bondy, Ed. CRC Press: Boca Raton, Florida.

Sandmeyer, E. 1981. Aromatic Hydrocarbons. In Clayton, G. D. and Clayton, F. E. (1981), *Patty's Industrial Hygiene and Toxicology.* New York: John Wiley & Sons.

Schwartz, E. 1987. Proportionate mortality ratio analysis of automobile mechanics and gasoline service station workers in New Hampshire. *American Journal of Industrial Medicine,* 12:91–99.

Seth, P. and Chandra, S. 1989. Neurotoxic effects of manganese. In Bondy Stephen. 1988. Metal neurotoxicity. CRC Press: Boca Raton, Florida.

Soderman, G. 1972. *Hereditas* 71(2):335. Found in Clayton, G. D., and Clayton, F. E. (1981), *Patty's Industrial Hygiene and Toxicology,* New York: John Wiley & Sons.

ORGANIC MERCURY TOXICITY

Organic mercury compounds were introduced into agricultural practice in Germany around 1915. They were used as liquid preparations for the treatment of seed grain, to prevent fungal disease before germination and during the growth of plants, fruits, and vegetables. Since that time, a wide variety of alkyl, alkoxyalkyl, and aryl compounds have been introduced (Ecobichon and Joy, 1982). Alkyl refers to a univalent group derived from the alkanes which contains one less hydrogen atom. Alkoxyalkyl refers to a combination of two alkyl groups and mercury. Aryl refers to a univalent group derived from the aromatic hydrocarbons which has a ring structure characteristic of benzene and its derivatives.

Chemistry

Mercury and its derivatives can be classified into inorganic ionic salts and organic salts, in which the mercury is bound covalently to at least one carbon atom (Ecobichon and Joy, 1982). Phenyl mercuric acetate (PMA) ($C_6H_5HgOOCCH_3$) is made by heating benzene with mercuric acetate (Windholz et al. 1983).

Toxicity

All forms of mercury are poisonous if absorbed. The poisonous effects of mercury are usually associated with the mercuric ion. Acute poisoning has been viewed as the major threat in the home and on the farm, but because mercury is a cumulative poison, subacute and chronic intoxications are also significant. (Gosselin et al., 1984).

An organic mercury compound, phenylmercuric acetate (PMA), has a toxicity rating of 5 (extremely toxic). The lethal oral dose for humans is 5 to 50 mg/kg; or for a 70 kg (150 pound) individual, a dose between 7 drops and one teaspoonful (tsp) would be fatal. The acute lethal dose is probably one half that of mercuric chloride. The LD50 in mice is 5 to 7 mg (as Hg/kg by parenteral routes and about 10 mg/kg by mouth). The oral LD50 of phenylmercuric acetate is reported to be 22 mg/kg in rats and 26 mg/kg in mice. Phenylmercuric acetate is easily absorbed through all portals, including intact skin (Gosselin et al., 1984).

Acute inorganic mercury toxicity signs and symptoms arise essentially from the mercuric cation. The acute symptoms generally result from the ingestion of large quantities of the agent. The symptoms include burning of the mouth and throat, extreme salivation, thirst, nausea, vomiting, severe gastrointestinal irritation with abdominal pain, bloody diarrhea, shock, loss of fluids and electrolytes, rapid and weak pulse, cardiac arrhythmias, clammy cold skin and pallor, peripheral vascular collapse, and slow breathing. Delayed toxicological signs may be observed some 2 to 7 days after the acute exposure and will include swelling of the salivary glands, persistent excessive salivation, metallic taste, stomatitis, soft spongy gums with loosened teeth showing the characteristic blue-black gum line caused by mercury-sulfhydiyl complexes. Oliguria is often present with anuria, uremia, albuminuria, hematuria, proteinuria, and acidosis. The classical picture of acute poisoning emerges as effects arising from two organ systems, the alimentary tract and the kidneys. The liver may also be affected, a central necrosis being observed. The above description is related only to the ingestion of large amounts of inorganic salts or possibly aryl- and alkoxyalkyl-mercurials which can be converted into mercuric ions. (Ecobichon and Joy, 1982).

Acute organic mercury intoxication results in motor and sensory nerve damage, which is irreversible in the case of severe alkylmercurial poisoning, and results in permanent brain damage. Even after acute exposure to toxic concentrations of alkylmercurials, several weeks or months may pass before the characteristic clinical signs appear (Ecobichon and Joy, 1982).

Acute intoxication, caused by inhalation of mercury vapor in high concentrations, was at one time common among those who extracted mercury from its ores. The condition is characterized by a metallic taste, nausea, abdominal pain, vomiting, diarrhea, headache, and sometimes albuminuria. After a few days, the salivary glands swell, stomatitis and gingivitis develop, and a dark line of mercury forms on the inflamed gums. The teeth may become loose, and ulcers may form on the lips and cheeks. In milder cases, recovery occurs within 10 to 14 days, but in others, poisoning of the chronic type may ensue, accompanied by muscular tremors and psychic disturbances (Wands, 1981).

Perhaps because some forms of organic mercury are so rapidly converted to inorganic mercury, these compounds do not appear to cross the blood-brain barrier in significant amounts. Thus, shortly after single exposures, the brains of laboratory animals contain much less mercury than do other organs and tissues; kidneys and liver accumulate the major burden. With time, the retained mercury is redistributed, so that the blood/brain concentration ratio falls toward 1.0. As with inorganic salts of mercury, repeated exposure to these organo-mercurials causes a slow but progressive increase in brain levels of mercury (Gosselin et al., 1984).

Chronic mercury toxicity continues to occur from both inorganic and organic mercury compounds. It may appear after a few weeks of exposure, or it may be delayed for much longer periods. Psychological and emotional disturbances are characteristic; the victim is often described as becoming excitable and irascible, especially when criticized. Other manifestations include loss of the ability to concentrate, with the patient becoming fearful, indecisive, or depressed, and complaining of headache, fatigue, weakness, loss of memory, and either drowsiness or insomnia. Objectively, the subject exhibits a fine tremor, and is unsteady in attempts to perform fine motions. The tremor may affect the hands, head, lips, tongue, or jaw. Writing is affected, letters being omitted or illegible. Other neurological disturbances include parasthesias, disturbances of taste or smell, neuralgia, and dermographism, a form of urticaria in which whealing occurs (at the site and in the configuration of an application of stroking, pressure, or friction) on the skin. (Wands, 1981).

Signs of renal disease are common; chronic nasal catarrh and epistaxis are not unusual. Salivation, gingivitis, and digestive disturbances are common. Stomatitis (inflammation of the mucous membrane of the mouth) is sometimes severe. Ocular lesions, such as amblyopia and scotomas occur, particularly from organic mercurials, narrowing the visual field. In general, symptoms from organic mercury exposure are confined to the nervous system. Most patients show slow recovery when removed from exposure (Wands, 1981).

Poisoning from the organic mercury compounds of industrial origin, the phenyl or methoxyethyl mercury compounds, is manifested by symptoms of fatigue, dyspnea, chest and abdominal pain, and vomiting. In some cases, gingivitis, dysarthria, motor weakness, and abdominal reflexes have been noted. In general, however, the signs and symptoms of aryl and methoxyethyl poisoning resemble those of inorganic mercury compounds (Wands, 1981).

The syndromes of chronic intoxication induced by inorganic mercury and by many organic mercurials are very similar, and are probably explained by the rapid metabolic breakdown of these mercurials to the mercuric ion. For example, studies on the fate and excretion of phenylmercuric acetate in rats, dogs, and chickens indicate that phenyl mercury is absorbed intact from many portals, transported largely in red blood cells, metabolized in the liver, and perhaps elsewhere, to release inorganic mercury, which in rats is excreted mostly in feces. Within 2 to 4 days, essentially all of the phenyl mercury was broken down. Hydroxylation of the phenyl ring was thought to precede rupture of the carbon-to-mercury bond; hydroxyphenyl mercury compounds decompose spontaneously in the presence of acid and cysteine or BAL (dimercaprol, an antidote) (Gosselin et al., 1984).

Upon ingestion, different inorganic mercurials will be absorbed at different rates related to their solubilities in water or gastrointestinal fluid. Depending upon the compound ingested, some 2% to 20% may be retained in the body, the bulk of the dose being excreted in the feces, with a small amount appearing in the urine. Inorganic mercury, on being absorbed into the bloodstream, is associated with the plasma proteins and cellular elements, and is likely to be excreted in the urine. The half-life of inorganic mercury in erythrocytes was 16 days in one study. The body half-life of ionic inorganic mercury in human volunteers was $42 +/- 3$ days (Ecobichon and Joy, 1982).

Organic mercurials have a different pattern of distribution and a considerably longer half-life. Organic mercurials (e.g., PMA) are more completely absorbed from the intestinal tract, an estimated 90% to 95% and 50% to 85% of alkyl- and arylmercurials being absorbed, respectively. In the blood, the alkylmercurials have a much greater affinity for erythrocytes. In man, the half-life of a typical organic mercurial, monomethylmercury, has been measured at 50 + / − 3 days in the body (Ecobichon and Joy, 1982).

In the general population, excluding those with known exposures, mercury concentrations are said to range from less than 0.005 to 0.07 ppm in whole blood and from less than 0.001 to 0.22 ppm (but only rarely above 0.05) in urine. Thus, an analytic determination of more than 0.1 ppm (10 mg/dl) in either blood or urine suggests an unusual exposure. Mercury accumulates in hair as the hair grows at its root; concentrations in newly formed hair average about 250 times greater than concurrent blood levels. Mean (or median) values of mercury in the hair of the general population range from 2 to 9 ppm. Although the intestinal tract is an important excretory route for mercury, apparently too few specimens of feces have been analyzed to establish normal limits (Gosselin et al., 1984).

A 39-year old farmer who had used no precautions in dusting oat seeds with phenylmercuric acetate over a period of 5 to 6 years, and who excreted large amounts of mercury in his urine, died of an apparently progressive neurologic disease resembling amyotrophic lateral sclerosis. Five other farmers similarly exposed were said to have various motor disabilities (Gosselin et al., 1984).

Uzell and Oler (in press) studied neuropsychological functioning and chronic low-level mercury exposure. They compared 13 female dental workers with elevated head mercury levels with 13 workers with no measurable mercury levels. Chronic subtoxic levels of inorganic mercury appeared to produce changes in short-term nonverbal recall and heightened distress, without alteration in other measured mental functions.

Clarkson and Marsh (1976) reviewed methylmercury exposure in man. Methylmercury poisoning affected primarily the nervous system, causing peripheral sensory changes, constriction of the visual field, ataxia, mental changes and death. The populations studied included 6000 cases in Iraq which were caused by contaminated grain, 88 sailors who were exposed to methylmercury by eating tuna, and 21 infants born with severe damage to the central nervous system at Minamata, Japan.

REFERENCES

Clarkson, T. W. and Marsh, D. O. 1976. The toxicity of methylmercury in man: Dose-response relationships in adult populations. In *Effects of Dose-Response Relationships in Toxic Metals*. G. F. Nordberg, Ed. Elsevier: Amsterdam.

Ecobichon, D. and Joy, R. 1982. *Pesticides and Neurological Disease*. CRC Press: Boca Raton, Florida.

Gosselin, R. E., Smith, R. P., and Hodge, H. C. 1984. *Clinical Toxicology of Commercial Products*. Williams & Wilkins: Baltimore.

Uzzell, B. P. and Oler, J. (in press). Chronic low-level mercury exposure and neuropsychological functioning. *J. of Clin. and Exper. Neuropsychol.*

Wands, R. C. 1981. Alkane materials. In Clayton, G. D. and Clayton, F. E. *Patty's Industrial Hygiene and Toxicology*, 3rd Ed., John Wiley & Sons: New York. pp. 3045–3052.

Windholz, M., Budavari, S., Blumetti, R. F., Otterbein, E. S. 1983. (Eds.) *The Merck Index*. Merck & Co.: Rahway, New Jersey.

ORGANOPHOSPHATE NEUROTOXICITY

Organophosphorus (OP) pesticides are among the most poisonous materials commonly used for pest control. In terms of toxic action, they are related to one another and to a group of chemical warfare agents known as nerve gas.

General Toxicology

Absorption to a dangerous degree can occur through any portal, including intact human skin. Most occupational accidents involving parathion and its chemical relatives are ascribed to dermal exposure. Such exposure is one tenth less toxic than exposure by inhalation. The rate of absorption varies directly with ambient temperature. Long-term sequela of acute poisonings are rare but are described: they tend to be neuropsychiatric disorders, peripheral neuropathies, or myopathies (Gosselin et al., 1984).

Organophosphates can be extremely toxic in minute amounts. Signs and symptoms may be vague and nonspecific rather than the commonly expected parasympathetic signs and symptoms. Intoxication has been mistaken for psychosis, chronic fatigue syndrome, GI illness or flu, and URI (upper respiratory tract infection) (Hodgeson, 1988).

A large number of cases of OP poisoning were reported in the countries which were the first to use OPs, including the United States. Poisoning was caused by ingestion, inhalation, and skin absorption. An undesirable property of many OPs is the narrow zone of toxic action (from onset of symptoms to death).

OPs are rapidly absorbed through the mucous membranes and skin. Chronic poisoning by OPs can lead to headache, weakness, decline of memory, quick fatigue, disturbed sleep, loss of appetite, and disorientation. Psychological disorders, nystagmus, trembling and other nervous system disorders, including neuritis, paresis, and paralysis can be seen in some cases (Medved and Kagan, 1983).

Acute Symptoms

The pharmacologic and toxicologic effects of OPs are probably largely caused by inhibition of acetylcholinesterase, resulting in excess accumulation of acetylcholine at cholinergic synapses. This overabundance initially stimulates and subsequently paralyzes cholinergic synaptic transmission in the CNS, somatic nerves, autonomic ganglia, parasympathetic nerve endings, and some sympathetic nerve endings (e.g., sweat glands).

The OPs are a closely related family of chemicals varying only in potency and latency before onset of symptoms. OPs may be absorbed by virtually any route. Onset of symptoms is most rapid following inhalation, and least rapid following percutaneous absorption, usually less than 12 hours.

The signs and symptoms may be classified into three categories: 1. muscarinic (parasympathetic) (SLUD: Salivation, lacrimation, urination, and defecation), trouble breathing; 2. nicotinic (autonomic ganglia and somatic motor) muscular fasciculation, weakness, areflexia, tachycardia, pallor, and hypertension; and 3. CNS (restlessness, emotional lability, headache, tremor, drowsiness, confusion, slurred speech, ataxia, generalized weakness, delirium, psychosis, coma, and depression of respiratory and cardiovascular centers).

Long-term sequelae include peripheral neuropathies, memory impairment, personality changes, depression, confusion, and thought disorders (Goldfrank et al., 1986).

General Chronic Neurotoxicity

Despite methodological shortcomings in many of the published studies, the following behavioral sequela of organophosphate insecticide poisoning have been found (Ecobichon and Joy, 1982):

1. Impaired vigilance and reduced concentration
2. Slowing of information processing and psychomotor speed
3. Memory deficit
4. Linguistic disturbance
5. Depression
6. Anxiety and irritability

Neurological lesions include unpleasant and long-lasting polyneuritis, flaccid paralysis, degeneration of the myelin sheaths and axons.

Epidemiologic and Experimental Studies of Neurotoxicity

A study performed under EPA contract by Savage et al. (1988) evaluated 100 individuals who had previously experienced acute poisoning from exposure to organophosphate pesticides. Each case was matched with a control, who had not had organophosphate poisoning, on the variables of age, sex, education, occupational class, socioeconomic status, race and ethnic background. Examinations were conducted blindly. Mean elapsed time from exposure was 9 years. No differences were found on physical examination, audiometric tests, ophthalmic tests, or on 28 standards clinical serum and blood chemistry evaluations, or EEGs. On neurological testing, no difference was found in state of consciousness, orientation, language, serial subtraction, numbers forwards, numbers backwards, or remote memory. Significantly more abnormalities were found in recent memory, abstraction and mood (depression). No differences were found in the motor system examination (23 components), sensory systems, or integrative components.

Neuropsychological examination found significantly more impairment on the Average Impairment Rating and the Halstead Impairment Index, including reduced IQ, all verbal IQ subscales, and some performance IQ subscales. Twice as many cases as controls had Halstead-Reitan Battery summary scores in the range of brain damage. MMPI found greater social anxiety, suspiciousness, and social stress among the cases. Self-rating of neuropsychological function areas found cases reporting more difficulty in 11 of 32 items. Relatives who rated the subjects found that the exposed individuals had more problems related to neuropsychological function, along with depression, irritability, social withdrawal, and confusions.

These sequela were sufficiently subtle that the clinical neurological examination, clinical EEG, and ancillary laboratory tests could not discriminate poisoned subjects from controls. In contrast, neuropsychological tests found that the poisoned subjects were significantly worse than controls on 4 of 5 summary measures (cerebral damage or dysfunction) and on 18 of 34 individual subtest scores. The major deficits were cognitive rather than sensory or motor functions as assessed by neurological examination, and appeared on tests of abilities that receive limited evaluation in the clinical neurological examination.

Sixteen cases of OP poisoning with psychiatric sequelae were seen by Gershon and Shaw (1961). They described a number of cases in their article. Case 9 was misdiagnosed as schizo-affective, and given 21 sessions of ECT. He was constantly tired, cranky, and irritable, could not do things as easily as before, and was "like a zombie." He stayed at home, sitting about the house and garden and did nothing. This pattern of behavior was reported to be different from his behavior prior to exposure.

Of 16 patients, 7 were misdiagnosed as depressives and 5 as schizophrenics. In all 16, memory and concentration were sufficiently disturbed to interfere seriously with work and reading ability.

The authors felt, based upon their studies and the studies reported below, that these insecticides activated a tendency towards depressive and schizophrenic reactions.

Dyflos was administered to 17 schizophrenics and 9 manic-depressives (Rowntree et al., 1950). Psychosis and florid symptoms were reactivated in the schizophrenics, while depression increased in the manic-depressives. Ten normal subjects "developed a very characteristic picture of depression, irritability, lassitude, and apathy, and they looked dejected and felt unhappy."

Results of neuropsychologic tests and computer-analyzed EEG indicated an association between chronic OP pesticide exposure and frontal lobe impairment (Korsik and Sato, 1977).

Case Reports of Neurotoxicity

A fascinating case report is presented by Bear et al. (undated). They found that both a 50 year old professor of medicine at a New England university, and his cat displayed extreme aggression following the application of a commercial tick powder containing carbaryl to his cat. The cat became super-aggressive, killing a large number of small animals, and the professor was in a rage most of the time. The aggression subsided following cessation of the pesticide use.

Five office occupants developed symptoms of organophosphate poisoning after application of chlorpyrifos (Dursban) and a carbamate pesticide (Bendocarb, 1%). The exterminator, contacted by telephone, assured them that their symptoms were unrelated to exposure and were probably caused by a virus (Hodgeson et al., 1986).

From a teaspoon of Diazenon on the genitals, a patient had severe OP reaction, including seizure and loss of consciousness (Halle and Sloas, 1986).

Schizophrenic psychosis or depressive illness may occur after obvious acute organophosphate intoxication or may follow chronic subliminal exposure. Joubert and Joubert (1988) calculated symptom incidence from the Gershom and Shaw study (1961), and compared the symptoms of one of their patients with the symptom incidence of Gershom and Shaw (1961):

Case 2	Gershom and Shaw's Series (%)
Loss of memory	50
Depression	44
Irritability	25
Headache	23
Fatigue	13

Regarding specific OPs, parathion had been considered the prototype of a nonneurotoxic cholinesterase inhibitor. However, a patient with delayed polyneuropathy following a suicide attempt was described (de Jager et al., 1981).

In general, Namba et al. (1971) discussed the long-term, persistent changes in peripheral and central nervous system function following OP exposure. See Chapter 5 for case studies of OP poisoning.

APPENDIX
THIMET

Thimet, an organophosphorous pesticide, is composed of 85% phorate (Thimet MC-85 Insecticide, American Cyanamid Company, Marketing Label 1/87). Phorate (Thimet) is closely related to demeton (a systemic pesticide which is highly toxic to mammals). An acute oral dose of LD50 in rats is 1 to 5 mg/kg (in contrast to malathion, 900 to 5800 mg/kg) (Matsumura, 1985).

Phorate has a toxicity rating of 6, the most hazardous rating given by Gosselin et al. (1984). This rating corresponds with the description "super toxic"; the probable oral *lethal* dose is "a taste (less than 7 drops)" (Gosselin et al. 1984).

According to the USSR toxicity rating system, Thimet is in the most toxic class of toxicity—extremely toxic. *Encyclopedia of Occupational Health and Safety*, 3rd Revised Ed., 1983, Chapter; Pesticides, organophosphorous.

A miscellaneous note: Impurities present in many commercial pesticides can potentiate the toxicity of parent compounds. A few impurities have recently been shown to be inherently toxic and produce acute, late acute, or delayed neurotoxic effects (Hollingshaus et al. 1983).

REFERENCES

Bear, D., Rosenbaum, J., and Norman, R. Undated. Case report: Aggression in cat and man precipitated by a cholinesterase inhibitor.

Ecobichon, D., and Joy, R. 1982. *Pesticides and Neurological Disease*. CRC Press: Boca Raton.

Gershon, S., and Shaw, F. H. 1961. Psychiatric sequelae of chronic exposure to organophosphorus insecticides. *Lancet*. June 24, 1961. pp. 1371–88.

Goldfrank, L. R., Bresnitz, E. A., Kirstein, R. H., and Howland, M. A. 1986. Organophosphates. In *Toxicologic Emergencies*. 3rd Ed. pp. 686–693.

Gosselin, R. E., Smith, R. P., and Hodge, H. C. 1984. *Clinical Toxicology of Commercial Products*. Williams & Wilkins: Baltimore, MD.

Halle & Sloas, 1987. Percutaneous organophosphate poisoning. *Southern Medical Journal*. 80(9):1179–81. September 1987.

Hodgeson, M. J. 1988. Diagnosis and management of organophosphate poisoning. *Internal Medicine* 9(4):77–87. April 1988.

Hodgeson, M. J., Block, G. D., and Parkinson, D. K. 1986. Organophosphate poisoning in office workers. *Journal of Occupational Medicine*, 28(6):434–37. June 1986.

Hollingshaus J. G., Eya, B., and Fukuto, R. 1983. Chemistry of neurotoxic organophosphorus compounds. *Neurotox.* 4(1):95–96.

de Jager et al, 1981. Polyneuropathy after massive exposure to parathion. *Neurol.* (NY) 21(5):603–605.

Joubert, J. and Joubert, P. H. 1988. Chorea and psychiatric changes in organophosphate poisoning: A report of 2 further cases. S.A.M.J. Vol 74. July 2, 1988.

Korsik, R. J. and Sato, M. M. 1977. Effects of chronic organic pesticide exposure on the central nervous system. *Clin. Toxicol.* 11(1):83–95.

Matsumura, Fumio. 1985. *Toxicology of Pesticides.* Plenum Press: New York.

Medved, L. I. and Kagan, J. S. 1983. Pesticides, organophosphorus. In *Encyclopedia of Occupational Health and Safety*, 3rd revised Ed. Parmeggiani, L. Ed. International Labor Organization: Geneva.

Namba, T., Nolte, C. T., Jackrel, J., and Grob, D. 1971. Poisoning due to organophosphate insecticides. *Am. J. of Medicine* 50:475–492.

Rowntree, D. W., Nevin, S., and Wilson, A. 1950. Experimental administration of OP in humans. *J. Neurol. Psychit.* 13:47. (Found in Gershon and Shaw, 1961.)

Savage, E. P., Keefe, T. J., Mounce, L. M., Heaton, R. K., Lewis, J. A., and Burcar, P. J. 1988. Chronic neurological sequela of acute organophosphate pesticide poisoning. *Archives of Environmental Health*, 43(1):38–45.

POLYCHLORINATED BIPHENYLS (PCBs)

Physical and Chemical Properties of Polychlorinated Biphenyls (PCBs)

PCBs comprise a class of nonpolar chlorinated hydrocarbons with a biphenyl nucleus in which any or all of the hydrogen atoms have been replaced by chlorine (NIOSH, 1986).

Commercial PCBs are generally mixtures of many different chlorinated biphenyls, according to specific operational specifications. The approximate chlorine content of PCB mixtures is as follows: Arochlors, 1221, (21%), 1016 (42%), 1242 (42%), 1254 (54%), and 1260 (60%); Kanechlors, 300 (43%), 400 (48%), and 500 (53%) (Clayton and Clayton, 1981).

Properties of PCBs including thermal stability, nonflammability, and dielectric capability resulted in their use in electrical capacitors and transformers. In transformers containing PCBs, the dielectric fluid generally consists of 60% to 70% PCBs and up to 40% chlorinated benzenes. Trade names of PCB askarels (the generic term used to refer to a broad class of nonflammable, synthetic, chlorinated hydrocarbon insulating liquids) formulated in the United States include Pyranol, Inerteese, and Noflamol. The volume of fluid in transformers ranges from 40 to 1,500 gallons. Small capacitors contain less than 3 pounds of PCBs while large capacitors contain more than 3 pounds. Electrical capacitors (small and large) contain nearly 100% PCBs (NIOSH, 1986).

Exposure Limits

In industry, exposure to PCBs is primarily dermal. Following both dermal and oral exposures to low doses, effects can be delayed for months (Clayton and

Clayton, 1981). PCBs are readily absorbed, but they are poorly metabolized, and they consequently accumulate in tissues (Finkel, 1983).

The threshold limit of chlorodiphenyl (42% Cl) on skin, adopted by the ACGIH (American Conference of Governmental Industrial Hygienists) was a TLV-TWA value of 2 mg/m^3. The adopted TLV-TWA value for chlorodiphenyl (54% Cl) on skin was 0.5 mg/m^3 and the tentative TLV-STEL value was 1 mg/m^3 (Clayton and Clayton, 1981).

OSHA promulgated its PEL of one milligram per cubic meter of air for chlorodiphenyl products containing 42% chlorine and .5 mg/m^3 for products containing 54% chlorine. These levels were thought to not cause liver injury in exposed workers (NIOSH, 1986).

NIOSH recommended that exposure to PCBs in the workplace be limited at or below the minimum reliable detectable concentration of 1 μg/m^3 (for a 40 hour week). The NIOSH recommended exposure limit (REL) was based on studies of adverse reproductive effects in experimental animals, and those studies have not demonstrated a level of exposure to PCBs that will not subject the worker to possible liver injury (NIOSH, 1986).

Work Hygiene

As a result of fire-related incidents involving PCB-containing electrical equipment, emergency response personnel, maintenance and clean-up workers, and building occupants may be at risk of exposure to PCBs, PCDFs, and PCDDs. The following NIOSH (1986) recommendations are intended to minimize worker exposure to these compounds. These recommendations focus primarily on PCB transformer fires.

Recognition of Potential Hazard. Emergency response personnel should be informed of the presence of PCB-containing electrical equipment and of the potential health hazards associated with exposure to emissions from such equipment. All workers should understand that exposure can occur through inhalation, ingestion, and skin absorption (by direct contact or by contact with contaminated surfaces, clothing, and equipment) and recognize that exposure to some of these compounds may result in long term effects.

Personal Protective Clothing. Outer protective garments should consist of a zippered coverall with attached hood and draw string, elastic cuffs, gloves, and closure boots. Such garments should be made of chemically resistant materials such as Saranax coated Tyvek or Victon coated Neoprene.

Respiratory Protection. Where a risk of airborne contaminants exists (soot), workers should wear a self-contained breathing apparatus with a full facepiece.

If no airborne PCBs can be detected, air purifying full facepiece respirators equipped with high efficiency particulate air filters and organic vapor cartridges should be used until final decontamination is completed.

Decontamination and Worker Protection Programs. Each stage of decontamination, such as gross decontamination and repetitive wash/rinse cycles, should be conducted separately, either by using different locations or by spacing in time. Personnel decontamination areas should be physically separated from the contaminated areas to prevent cross-contact and should be arranged in order of decreasing level of contamination.

All reusable clothing and equipment should be grouped according to perceived degree of contamination (i.e., high, moderate, and low) and thoroughly cleaned. Reusable clothing and equipment should be analyzed for residual contamination before reuse or storage.

Medical Surveillance. A medical surveillance program should be established to prevent (or to attempt to detect at an early stage) adverse health effects in workers resulting from exposure to PCBs or related compounds. Medical and work histories, including previous exposure to PCBs and other toxic agents, should be taken for each worker prior to job placement, and this information should be updated periodically. The responsible physician should be provided with information concerning the adverse health effects from exposure to PCBs and related compounds, and an estimate of the worker's potential exposure, including any available workplace sampling results and a description of all protective clothing or equipment the worker may be required to use (NIOSH, 1986).

An Italian study of electrical workers concluded that in the plants studied, absorption of PCBs occured mainly through the skin, so the commonly used method to assess industrial exposure to atmospheric PCBs is not sufficient to give complete information on the exposure level of the workers. Guidelines for preventing undue exposure in industry must consider protection against skin absorption (Maroni et al., 1981).

Since 1977, government regulations in the United States have prohibited the manufacture of transformers and capacitors containing PCBs as dielectric fluids. However, it has been estimated that over 150,000 tons of PCBs are present in capacitors and transformers still in use. In 1978, laboratory experiments demonstrated that pyrolysis of PCBs at high temperatures ($200\,^{\circ}C$ to $600\,^{\circ}C$) could result in the formation of significant amounts of the more toxic polychlorinated dibenzofurans (PCDFs) (O'Keefe et al., 1985).

Despite the ban, the danger of significant exposures remains for particular occupational groups. Utility workers, for example, may experience sporadic but potentially massive exposures when cleaning up spills, or when servicing or dismantling transformers and capacitors that still contain PCB fluid. Electricians, appliance service workers, and firefighters also may have continued occupational exposure (Letz, 1982).

General Toxicity

In all animal species that have been studied, PCBs have a very low acute toxicity. They are readily absorbed across biological membranes, poorly metabolized and only very slowly eliminated (Letz, 1982).

Surveys in various geographical areas have found detectable residues in blood, fat, and mother's milk. Measurable levels of PCBs are typically found in greater than 50% of subjects tested, with maximum blood levels generally less than 20 ppb. The levels reported from adipose tissue are typically somewhat higher, in the range of 1 to 2 ppm. Residues of PCBs in human milk have ranged from 40 to 100 ppb in whole milk (Letz, 1982).

In general, the higher the exposure levels, the higher the blood concentration of PCBs; and the higher the environmental concentration and/or longer the period of exposure, the longer the blood levels of PCBs remain elevated (Letz, 1982).

A cross-sectional study of 120 male workers was conducted to determine polychlorinated biphenyl (PCB) absorption and the presence of potentially related clinical and metabolic abnormalities. Three exposure categories, *exposed*, *nominally exposed*, and *nonexposed*, were defined. The PCB levels among the exposed group showed a clear elevation when compared with those of either the nominally exposed or nonexposed group. The average plasma PCB level (33.4 ppb) of the exposed group was more than twice that of either the nominally exposed group (14.2 ppb) or the nonexposed group (12.0 ppb). The discrepancy in fat PCB level for the exposed group was 5.6 ppm, more than three times that of either the nominally exposed (1.4 ppm) or the nonexposed group (1.3 ppm). The subjects in the two exposed groups were older than those in the nonexposed group. The average ages were 41.4 years for the exposed group, 37.2 years for the nominally exposed group, and 30.7 years for the nonexposed group. The average lengths of employment were 17 years, 3 years 9 months, and 4 years 3 months, respectively. The differences in age and length of employment were significant (Chase et al., 1982).

The PCB levels observed in the subjects in the nominally and the nonexposed groups coincide with reported normal ranges in nonexposed populations for both plasma (<30 ppb) and fat (<2.0 ppm) PCB levels. In contrast, the findings of significantly elevated plasma and fat levels among those in the exposed group support the premise that the occupational exposure to PCBs can lead to increased PCB absorption and retention. This relationship is further strengthened by the demonstrated correlation between length of employment and PCB levels. This association was stronger with fat than with plasma PCB levels, suggesting that fat levels are a more precise index of cumulative exposure (Chase et al. 1982).

A Japanese study of PCBs in patients with Yusho disease revealed that PCB levels declined with time. Several years after the outbreak, the average concentrations of PCBs in the adipose tissue, liver, and blood of patients were 1.9 ppm, 0.08 ppm, and 6.7 ppb, respectively, and only two times higher than those of control patients, indicating that most of the PCBs ingested by the patients had been eliminated (Masuda and Yoshimura, 1984).

Neurotoxicity of PCBs and Dibenzofurans

Fischbein et al. (1979) studied 326 capacitor manufacturing workers who had been exposed to dielectric fluids containing PCBs. Ninety percent were employed for more than 5 years, and 40% for 20 years or longer. Neurologic symptoms were cited by 39% of the males and 58% of the female workers; the symptoms included headache, dizziness, depression, sleep problems, nervousness, fatigue, and memory loss.

Thirty-five patients out of the 2,000 PCB-poisoned cases that occured in central Taiwan (Yu-Cheng Disease) in 1978 were studied in 1980, one to two years after ingesting contaminated cooking oil (Chia and Chu, 1984). Mean blood PCB concentration was 34.6 ppb, compared with less than 4 ppb in normal control subjects at the hospital where the study was done. Neurological manifestations included clinical peripheral sensory neuropathy in 33%, headache in 37%, dizziness in 34%, paresthesia (an abnormal spontaneous sensation, such as burning, pricking, tickling or tingling) and numbness in the distal part of the limbs in 66%, hypoesthesia (diminution of sensitivity) or hypalgesia (diminished sensitivities to pain) in the distal part of limbs in 37%, absent or sluggish deep tendon reflexes in 17%, and EEG abnormalities (paroxysmal bilateral slow waves, occasionally mixed with sharp waves or spikes in the frontotemporal region) in 22% (these cases had no history of epilepsy).

Mean NCVs of the ulnar, radial, tibial, and sural nerves were slower than those of the control group. There were 16 patients whose motor NCV and/or sensory NCV (one, two, or three nerves) were below normal. In 23 patients with clinical signs of peripheral neuropathy, the slowed NCVs were found as follows: ulnar nerve, 3 cases; tibial nerve, 5 cases; radial nerve, 4 cases; and the sural nerve, 5 cases. However, in 12 patients without clinical peripheral neuropathy, NCVs were also slow. No statistical differences were found comparing those with and without clinical peripheral neuropathy. Sensory NCV was reduced in about half of the cases and motor NCV was reduced in about one-third of the cases, which suggests that PCB poisoning can affect both sensory and motor NCV.

Overall, 89% had one or more neurological symptoms and signs. The authors attributed widespread neural dysfunction to the high fat solubility of PCBs, and their consequent distribution to adipose tissues or tissues with a high lipid content, e.g., the myelin sheath of the peripheral nerve.

Seppalainen et al. (1985) performed serial NCV assessments (two and six months post-exposure) on 16 men exposed to PCBs and related contaminants from a capacitor accident. The highest blood PCB concentrations were found three days after the explosion; PCB levels decreased to the baseline within one to two months.

A reversible impairment of the peripheral nerves was noted mainly in the distal portions of the sensory nerves, where NCV and the amplitude of the sensory action potentials had decreased. The authors noted that this pattern of findings is typical of toxic distal axonopathy, in which there is symmetrical axonal degeneration beginning distally in long and large peripheral nervous system tracts. However, at six months post-exposure, only the sural and distal ulnar sensory NCVs were slightly slower than control nerves.

A number of animal studies have evaluated the neurotoxicity of PCBs. Seegal et al. (1986; 1986b) found alterations in brain chemistry in the mature mammalian nervous system following brief exposure to PCBs. Bowman et al. (1978) found that PCBs can induce behavior deficits in monkeys.

Singer (1988) reported a neuropsychological evaluation of a PCB toxicity incident. A number of workers were employed by a metal salvage company that was stripping copper coils from used electrical transformers. PCB contamination was found at the site, which became the focus of federal and state remedial clean-up efforts. The salvage process caused the men to become soaked with transformer fluid. The exposure occurred over a three-year period. Additional exposure to smoke occured from burning transformer fluid.

One to two years after the exposure began, the subject of this study became impotent, irritable, and began losing his temper over trivial matters. He developed concentration and short-term memory difficulties, fatigue, and had trouble figuring out mechanical problems. He also developed muscle spasms in the back, neck, and legs, and periodic numbness in his legs. The PCB level in his fat was 1.65 ppm two years after the exposure.

Prior to exposure, the subject was apparently in excellent health and had superior cognitive and memory skills. He was director of maintenance for a major U.S. airline, European division, and at the time of exposure was vice-president of the salvage company.

The tests that were administered included the Wechsler Adult Intelligence Scale, Revised (WAIS-R), Benton Visual Retention Test, the Wechsler Memory Scale: Logical Memory, Grooved Pegboard Test, Trailmaking (A, B), malingering tests, and conduction velocity and amplitude tests of the median motor, median sensory, and sural nerves, bilaterally.

Upon repeated examinations, deficits were found on the Digit Span, Block Design and Digit Symbol Subtests of the WAIS-R, Visual Retention Test, and the Logical Memory Tests, indicating functional deficits in short-term visual and auditory memory, delayed verbal memory, and visuo-spatial perception. Sural nerve responses were abnormal, bilaterally, and right median sensory response was borderline. This pattern of symptoms and deficits is consistent with chronic human nervous system dysfunction from PCB transformer fluid. Similar results were found in two of three co-workers.

Another worker at the same site was studied, and the results are reported in Chapter 7.

Jackson (1985) reported a case of neuropsychiatric manifestations of chronic PCB intoxication. A man exposed for 8 years to PCB-containing transformer fluid (Arochlor 1260) had subtle, long-term cognitive impairment in the absence of major neurologic findings. Symptoms included diminished intellectual abilities, decreased libido, and depression.

REFERENCES

Bowman, B. E., Heironimus, M. P., and Allen, J. R. 1978. Correlation of PCB body burden with behavioral toxicology in monkeys. *Pharmacol. Biochem. and Behavior* 9:49–56.

Chase, K. H. et al. 1982. Clinical and metabolic abnormalities associated with occupational exposure to polychlorinated biphenyls (PCBs). *Journal of Occupational Medicine* 24(2):109–114.

Chia, L.-G. and Chu, F.-L. 1984. Neurologic studies on polychlorinated biphenyl (PCB)-poisoned patients. *Am. J. of Ind. Med.* 5:117–126.

Clayton, G. D. and Clayton, F. E. 1981. *Patty's Industrial Hygiene and Toxicology.* 3rd Ed., Volume 2B, John Wiley & Sons: New York. pp. 3654–3669.

Finkel, A. J. 1983. *Hamilton and Hardy's Industrial Toxicology.* 4th Ed., Wright PSG: Boston, MA. pp. 238–240.

Fischbein, A. et al. 1979. Clinical findings among PCB capacitator-exposed manufacturing workers. *Am. N.Y. Acad. Sci.* 320:703–715.

Gosselin, R. E. et al. 1984. Clinical Toxicology of Commercial Products. 5th Ed., Williams & Wilkins: Baltimore, MD. Section II, pp. 171–172.

Jackson, J. E. 1985. Neuropsychological manifestations of chronic PCB intoxication. *Vet. Hum. Toxicol.* 28(4):299.

Letz, G. 1982. *The Toxicology of PCBs.* Hazard Evaluation System and Information Service, Department of Health Services: Berkeley, CA.

Maroni, M. et al. 1981. Occupational exposure to polychlorinated biphenyls in electric workers. I. Environmental and blood polychlorinated biphenyls concentrations. *Brit. J. Indus. Med.* 38:49–54.

Masuda, Y. and Yoshimura, H. 1984. Polychlorinated biphenyls and dibenzofurans in patients with Yusko and their toxicologic significance: A review. *Am. J. Ind. Med.* 5:31–34.

Murai, Y. and Kuroiwa, Y. 1971. Peripheral neuropathy in chlorobiphenyl poisoning. *Neurology* 21:1173–1176.

NIOSH. 1986. *Polychlorinated Biphenyls (PCB's): Potential Health Hazards from Electrical Equipment Fires or Failures.* Central Intelligence Bulletin 45, National Institute for Occupational Safety and Health, DHHS (NIOSH) Publication No. 86-111. February 24, 1986.

O'Donoghue, J. L. (Ed.) 1985. *Neurotoxicity of Industrial and Commercial Chemicals.* Vol. 1. CRC Press: Boca Raton, FL. p. 125.

O'Keefe, P. W. et al. 1985. Chemical and biological investigations of a transfer accident at Binghamton, New York. *Environmental Health Perspectives* 60:201–209.

Reggiani, R. and Bruppacher, R. 1985. Symptoms, signs and findings in humans exposed to PCBs and their derivatives. *Environmental Health Perspectives* 60:225–232.

Seegal, R. F., Brosch, K. O., and Bush, B. 1986a. Polychlorinated biphenyls produce regional alterations of dopamine metabolism in rat brain. *Toxicology Letters* 30:197–202.

Seegal, R. F., Brosch, K. O., and Bush, B. 1986b. Regional alterations in sertonin metabolism induced by oral exposure of rats to polychlorinated biphenyls. *Neurotoxicology* 7(1):155–166.

Seegal, R. F., Brosch, K. O., and Bush, B. 1985. Polychlorinated biphenyls produce regional alterations of norephinephrine concentrations in adult rat brain. *Neurotoxicology* 6(3):13–24.

Seegal, R. F., Brosch, K. O., and Bush, B. 1985. Oral dosing of rats with polychlorinated biphenyls increases urinary homovanillic acid production. *J. of Toxicol. Environ. Health* 15:575–586.

Seppalainen, A. M. et al. 1985. Reversible nerve lesions after accidental polychlorinated biphenyl exposure. *Scand. J. Work. Environ. Health* 11:91–95.

Singer, R. 1988. Methodology of forensic neurotoxicity evaluation: PCB case. *Toxicology,* 49:403–408.

RADIATION NEUROTOXICITY

Radiation Physics. Matter is composed of atoms, containing neutrons, protons, and electrons (Miller, 1972). The heavy particles, neutrons and protons, can change states into one another. When the changeover within the nucleus of the atom occurs spontaneously, the nucleus is said to be radioactive, or unstable. Three kinds of radiations are emitted: alpha rays, which are stopped by a sheet of paper; beta rays, which are high speed electrons, which can be stopped by a few centimeters of flesh; and gamma rays, which are high energy photons, such as X-rays.

Nuclear radiation results in ionization, the stripping of one or more bound electrons from an atom or molecule (Holahan, 1987). Charged particles directly disrupt (ionize) chemical bonds and thus produce chemical and biological changes. Electromagnetic radiation is indirectly ionizing since it does not itself produce any chemical or biological change. Rather, it transfers kinetic energy into the material through which it passes, and produces secondary charged particles (electrons) that can induce subsequent chemical and biological changes.

Regardless of the type of ionizing radiation, the final common event is the ejection or excitation of bound orbital electrons.

Measurement of Radiation. A roentgen (R) is a unit of exposure that is used for X-ray and gamma radiation. Therapeutic radiation is usually measured in Rad or Gray (Gy), which are units of energy, radiation absorbed dose, and denotes the amount of energy divided by matter or mass of body tissue, or energy per tissue. One Gy equals 100 rad, and one R equals 1 rad in tissue.

Biological Mechanisms of Radiation. Ionizing radiation damages cells by stripping orbital electrons from atoms (Spivak, 1984). The ejected electrons then dissipate their energy by ionizing other molecules within the cell. Ionization creates free radicals, which can become involved in a variety of chemical reactions that can be deleterious to critical intracellular molecules.

The deposition of energy by ionizing radiation in cells causes hydrogen bonds to sunder, molecular degradation or breakage, and intramolecular and intermolecular cross-linking (Holahan, 1987). This leads to disorganization within the cell and within the DNA, the cell reproductive organizer. Damage to cells can be classified as lethal, sublethal, and potentially lethal.

Tissues differ in their sensitivity to radiation. Cells that are most sensitive to radiation are those still capable of replication (Caveness, 1980). The sensitive cells of the central nervous system (the brain and spinal cord) include glial cells (see Appendix 1 for a description of glial cell function) and endothelial cells. Endothelial cells (cells that line the blood vessels) are critical for maintaining the blood-brain barrier, which protects the brain from many toxic substances. These cells also control optimum ionic gradients. The orderly flow of fluids and solutes through the extracellular spaces and their return through the cerebral and vascular system depends upon intact endothelial cells. When these cells are damaged, the functioning and survival of the dependent neurons is jeopardized.

Radiation causes damage to the DNA within the cells. This damage interferes with the cells' ability to replicate, repair damage, and support the dependent neurons.

Regional irradiation of the brain with a single exposure may lead to initial increase in capillary permeability with marked tissue swelling, edema or swelling extending from the irradiated area (remote edema), an increase in cerebral-spinal fluid pressure, blindness, depression of the visual evoked response, changes in the EEG, a decrease in regional cerebral blood flow, and incomplete healing.

Whole brain irradiation, in fractionated exposure from 4,000 to 8,000 rads, 1000 rads per week, 200 rads per day, was studied in monkeys. The hallmark lesion was a minute focus of necrosis widely scattered throughout the forebrain white matter, appearing in one half to two years. Accompanying or perhaps preceding the discrete areas of necrosis were a variety of vascular abnormalities, notably affecting the endothelial cells.

Purpose of Radiation Treatment for Tumors. Radiation is given to kill tumor cells. Because the tumor cells are often replicating faster than non-tumor cells, they are more susceptible to radiation effects than many other organs. There is a cost benefit ratio to be considered with radiation therapy: a higher dosage may kill more tumor cells, but will also injure non-tumor cells, while a lower dose may be less effective in eradicating tumor cells.

Classification. Adverse effects of brain irradiation for cancer treatment may be divided into three groups according to time of appearance (Sheline, 1980). These are 1. *acute reactions*, which occur during the course of irradiation; 2. *early delayed reactions*, which are usually transient and appear from a few weeks to a few months after irradiation; and 3. *late delayed reactions*, with onset from several months to several years after exposure.

Delayed Damage. Delayed damage to the central nervous system (CNS) due to X-ray radiation was described in 1930 and has been studied since (Holdorff, 1978). In 1934, researchers distinguished between early and late reactions. The latter were described as chronic progressive encephalopathy. A dose-response effect of radiation damage to the CNS was observed as early as 1938, when researchers warned against increasing focal doses above 4,000 to 5,000 rads.

Latency. Although the latency period between the end of irradiation and the occurrence of clinical symptoms of delayed radiation damage varies from months to years, shorter latency periods have been reported, such as 8 to 10 weeks. Brain stem lesions have in general a shorter symptom-free period than lesions of the hemispheres.

Tolerance Dose. The tolerance dose of the brain has been given as 4,000 $\pm$ 1,000 rads in the case of a 100 cm^2 field, fractionated into 30 to 35 days.

Morphology of Early Changes. Single exposures to high doses—if they do not cause death—give rise to acute cerebral radiation necrosis of all tissue elements. Acute inflammatory changes occur in the meninges and blood vessels and selected damage to the granular layer of the cerebellar cortex also takes place. These early changes manifest during the first hours and days after high dosage exposure. Moderate dosage radiation, such as occurs in fractionated radiation treatment for cancer, gives rise to fewer early changes.

Other clinical changes that have been observed include reduction in the blood-brain barrier, inflammation, edema, astroglia (degenerative changes in the astrocytes, one of the large neuroglia cells of the nervous system), oligodendroglia (degeneration of one of the three types of glial cells in the CNS, this one forming the myelin sheath of the nerve fibers), damage to the nerve cells (with higher doses), and total necrosis (cell death from irreversible damage).

Morphology of Delayed Changes.   If delayed changes occur after a silent period, during which no obvious alterations have been apparent, a progresive degeneration is indicated. The morphological symptoms include initially selective damage of the white matter, followed by total necroses. Even during the latency period, fundamental changes are present.

Clinical Picture of Radiation Damage.   Early reactions include changes in EEG (even at low doses), increase in intracranial pressure, cerebral edema and transient neurological symptoms. Delayed reactions can include seizures, disruption in sensory, motor, thinking or any faculties of the brain, dementia, etc. (Holdorff, 1978).

Behavioral Aspects of Ionizing Radiation.   Exposure to ionizing radiation has multiple effects on the brain and behavior, depending upon dose (Hunt, 1987). In some cases, the effect is transient, but in others it is permanent. The effects include incapacitation, problems with motor performance, decision making, short-term memory, visual discrimination, and other effects. Irradiated monkeys tended to focus their attention narrowly on the task at hand. Experimental data suggests that well-learned tasks may be accomplished, but attention to new detail was diminished.

Neuropsychological Effects of Radiation to the Brain for Cancer Treatment

The psychiatric manifestations of cancer therapy on the central nervous system can vary from mild focal impairment of intellectual functioning to the global impairment of toxic psychosis or dementia (Silberfarb and Oxman, 1988). Since the problem of cognitive impairment covers a spectrum ranging from subtle to dramatic, the impairment is often missed by the clinician when it is "mild." The subtle loss of cognitive function can be measured with objective tests. Impaired cognitive function may be correlated with a relative slowing of the EEG. Neuropsychological testing to determine the possible effects of radiation on brain function in cancer patients receiving radiation is recommended. Radiation therapy, both alone and in combination with chemotherapy, has been reported to produce neurotoxicity.

Radiation damage to the brain was reviewed from a neuropsychiatric perspective by McMahon and Vahora (1986). Neuropsychiatric manifestations of late-delayed reactions include IQ and reading deficits in children, and progressive deterioration of cognitive functions in adults. The cases of two women who developed radiation necrosis were presented. Cognitive and affective symptoms were a prominent part of the clinical picture.

The long-term neurotoxicity associated with cancer treatment of the CNS was first recognized in the 1970s (Kramer and Moore, 1989). Since then, the deleterious effects of CNS treatment on brain function and structure have become a major concern to those working in the field of clinical oncology. Cognitive deficits and brain abnormalities are frequently reported in studies of children's cancer therapies.

Patients with leukemia receiving chemotherapy alone were compared with patients receiving chemotherapy and cranial irradiation (Rowland et al., 1984). Children whose CNS therapy included cranial radiation performed significantly less well than the nonirradiated children on measures of general intelligence (IQ) and school achievement (word recognition, spelling and arithmetic). This study implicated radiation as the most significant cause of reduced cognitive function in the children studied.

The intellectual deficits reported in studies of leukemia survivors are usually diffuse in nature, but specific impairments have also been reported (Kramer and Moore, 1989), namely deficits in visual memory integration, memory dysfunction, verbal learning deficits, impairment of verbal and visuospatial learning measures, and attentional deficits.

Children with medulloblastoma receive surgery and whole-brain radiation (Kramer and Moore, 1989). In studies of these patients, significant intellectual impairment has been reported frequently. For example, in one study 89% of these patients had IQ scores below 90, as compared with 58% of their cerebellar astrocytoma control group, who did not receive whole-brain irradiation. In another study, brain tumor patients receiving whole brain irradiation showed a highly significant decline in IQ scores between 6 and 48 months after treatment, whereas patients receiving focal radiation or no radiation demonstrated a stable IQ during the same period. Intellectual impairment seems to be increased with increasing dosages of radiation. The highest dosage level studies were up to 4,000 rads.

Neuroimaging techniques such as CAT scans and MR have consistently indicated that CNS cancer treatments can result in alterations of brain structure (Kramer and Moore, 1989). Radiation appears to cause periventricular hypodensity, a decrease in white matter, and other white matter changes. White matter pathology has been documented by neuroimaging techniques as well as animal studies of delayed radiation injury. Vascular changes have been documented in animals after low to moderate doses of radiation. Cranial irradiation may damage the tight junctions formed by the endothelial cells of the blood-brain barrier.

A neuropsychological test battery was administered in an adult with mental deterioration following cancer treatment, which included radiation (Kelly, 1988). Two patterns of neuropsychological deficits occurred simultaneously: a lateralized form corresponding with the tumor and surgery, and a diffuse dementiform pattern. The authors proposed that radiation caused the diffuse dementiform pattern. As discussed by the authors in their review of the scientific literature, irradiation injuries occur even when dosages are delivered under conditions and limits regarded as safe.

Regarding injuries occurring under "normal" radiotherapy dosage conditions (Marks, 1981), the risk of radionecrosis increased with increasing doses, but the risk was not correlated with time, fractionation, or larger field size. Radiotherapy applied too quickly after cranial surgery may increase the risk of radiation necrosis because the edema from the surgery appears to lower the resistance of brain tissue to radiation (Kelly et al., 1988).

Brain atrophy and dementia was found to follow radiation therapy for brain tumors (Asai et al., 1987). Radiation induced atrophy was observed in 51 of 91 patients (56%) and dementia in 23 of 47 (49%). These conditions occurred more frequently in aged and whole-brain irradiated patients. Radiation induced brain atrophy and dementia appeared 2 to 3 months after the completion of radiation therapy.

In a study of 15 cases of whole-brain radiation, 4000 to 5000 rads, in 180 to 200 fractions (Mechanick et al., 1986), dysfunction that preceded CAT-scan evidence of damage, and which preceded the onset of dementia was found. Fourteen patients displayed symptoms reflecting disturbances of personality, libido, thirst, appetite, or sleep. Seven patients developed cognitive abnormalities. Cortical atrophy was present in 50% of cases and third ventricular dilation in 58%. The authors concluded that hypothalamic dysfunction, heralded by endocrine, behavioral, and cognitive impairment, represents a common, subtle form of radiation damage.

Severe encephalopathy ensued in five patients within hours of receiving their initial dose of cranial irradiation (Oliff et al., 1978). Neurological findings included cranial-nerve palsies, seizures, ataxia, depressed consciousness, and increased intra-cranial pressure. Chemotherapy may have contributed to the findings.

Data from a large number of cancer patients was analyzed for radiation necrosis (Edwards and White, 1980). Ninety-two cases were found and analyzed. Various types of brain impairment occurred. The "early" delayed radiation necrosis syndrome was studied. "Early" radiation effects occurred in 25% of the patients, within between two weeks and three months of completion of therapy, with headache, confusion, and lethargy. Others have found that radiotherapy can provoke psychopathology and mental disorder (Popova, 1977).

APPENDIX
GLIAL CELLS

The tissues of the central nervous system are built with two main types of cells: neurons and glial cells (Somjen, 1987). Glial cells (neuroglia) connect neurons. They are of ectodermal origin. They also convey nutritive substances from blood to neurons. Glial cells are involved in the repair of neurons, and fill spaces vacated by neurons. Glial cells also insulate nerve cells and nerve fibers to prevent undesired cross-talk, and they form a protective filter around capillaries, keeping neurotoxic substances from entering the brain. They also remove metabolic waste from the brain, depositing it in the bloodstream.

There are three types of gila: astrocytes (astroglia), oligocytes (oligodendroglia), and microcytes (microglia). The main function of microglia is the removal of dead cells and other debris by phagocytosis. The main function of the oligocytes is the formation of myelin sheaths around central axons. Astrocytes proliferate after dead neurons have been cleared away, and form the scars of the brain.

Glial cells preseve homeostasis of the interstitial fluid of the central nervous system, by transporting materials to and from neurons and capillaries, and by preserving the pH of brain fluid. Astrocytes also synthesize some neurotransmitters.

REFERENCES

Asai, A. et al. 1987. Subacute brain atrophy induced by radiation therapy of malignant brain tumors. *Gan No Rinsho* 6/33(7):753–61.

Caveness, W. 1980. Experimental observations: Delayed necrosis in normal monkey brain. In *Radiation Damage to the Nervous System*, Gilbert and Kagan Eds. Raven Press: NY.

Edwards, M. and White, C. 1980. Treatment of radiation necrosis. In *Radiation Damage to the Nervous System*, Gilbert and Kagan Eds. Raven Press: NY.

Holahan, E. 1987. Cellular radiation biology. In *Military Radiobiology*, Conklin and Walker Eds. Academic Press: San Diego.

Holdorff, B. 1978. Radiation damage to the brain. In *Handbook of Clinical Neurology*, Vol. 23, pp. 639–664. Elsevier/North Holland: NY.

Hunt, W. A. 1987. Effects of ionizing radiation on behavior. In *Military Radiobiology*, Conklin and Walker Eds. Academic Press: San Diego.

Kelly, M. A. et al. 1988. Suspected late onset radionecrosis. Paper presented at the Eighth Annual Meeting of the National Academy of Neuropsychologists, Orlando, November 4, 1988.

Kramer, J. and Moore, I. M. 1989. Late effects of cancer therapy on the central nervous system. *Sem. in Oncol. Nurs.* 5(1):22–28.

Marks, J. E. et al. 1981. Cerebral radionecrosis: Incidence and risk in relation to dose, time, fractionation and volume. *Int. J. Radiation Oncology Biol. Phys.* 7:243–252.

McMahon, T. and Vahora, S. 1986. Radiation damage to the brain: Neuropsychiatric aspects. *Gen. Hosp. Psychiat.* 8(6):437–441.

Mechanick, J. I. et al. 1986. Hypothalamic dysfunction following whole brain radiation. *J. Neurosurg.* 65(4):490–94.

Miller, F. 1972. *College Physics*, Harcourt Brace Jovanovich: New York.

Oliff, A. et al. 1978. Acute encephalopathy after initiation of cranial irradiation for meningeal leukemia. *Lancet* 2(8079):13–15.

Owens, A. H. and Colvin, M. 1984. Neoplastic disease: Principles of management. *The Principles and Practice of Medicine*, 21st Ed. Harvey et al. Eds. Appleton-Century-Crofts: Norwalk, CT.

Popova, M. S. 1977. Effect of irradiation on the character of mental disorders observed in patients subjected to surgery on account of laryngeal neoplasms. *Zh. Neuropatol. Psikhiatr.* 77(2):262–6.

Rowland, J. H., Glidewell, O. J., and Sibley, R. F. 1984. Effects of different forms of central nervous system prophylaxis on neuropsychological function in childhood leukemia. *J. Clin. Oncol.* 2:1327–1335.

Sheline, G. 1980. Irradiation injury of the human brain. In *Radiation Damage to the Nervous System*, Gilbert and Kagan Eds. Raven Press: NY.

Silberfarb, P. and Oxman, T. 1988. The effects of cancer therapies on the central nervous system. *Adv. Psychosom. Med.* 18:13–25.

Somjen, G. 1987. Glial cells function. *Encyclopedia of Neuroscience*, Adelman, G. Ed. Vol. 1, p. 465. Birkhauser: Boston.

Spivak, J. L. 1984. Electrical and radiation injury. *The Principles and Practice of Medicine*, 21st Ed. Harvey et al. Eds. Appleton-Century-Crofts: Norwalk, CT.

INDEX

Accidents, 30
Aging and neurotoxicity, 29–33
Alar, 34–36
Alzheimer's disease, 26–27, 30–33
    liability and, 86
Ammonia, 149–152
Arsenic, 74
Asbestos, 81

Baygon, 109–114
Behavioral toxicology, 44–55
Benzene, 152–157
Biological monitoring, 41–45
    legal aspects of, 89–91
Blood analysis, 42

Cadmium, 181–182
Carbamates, 109–114
Carbon monoxide, 158–160
Causation, legal, 83
Chemicals, neurotoxic, 8–24
Chlordane, 22–23
    regulation of, 164–165
    toxicity of, 160–166
Chlorpyrifos, 109–114
Civil suits, 81–87
Computer assisted tomography (CAT scan),
    44
Construction workers, case reports, 109–114,
    139–143
Copper ore, 24

DDT, 21
Deficit measurement paradigm, 54–55, 66
Degreasing worker, case report, 94–99
Dementia, 29–33. *Also see* Alzheimer's
    disease
Dursban, 109–114

Electroencephalogram (EEG), 55
Employer's dilemma, 89–91

Evoked potential, 55–60
    auditory, 56
    brain, 55–57
    sensory, 56–57
    somatosensory, 56
    visual, 56

Fat biopsy, 42
Fishermen, 147–131
Formaldehyde, 23, 35
    case reports, 132–148
    sources of, 147–148, 166–178
    toxicity of, 166–178

Gasoline, 1, 16–19, 33, 178–183
Government regulation, 33–36

Hair analysis, 43
Headache, 6–7
Heptachlor toxicity, 160–166
Herbicides, 23, 74
Hydrogen sulfide
    case report, 147–131
    neurotoxicity of, 131

Indoor pollution, 82

Lead, 1–2, 45, 74
    case report, 122–126
    organic, 180–181
Legal aspects of neurotoxicity, 80–81
Liability
    absolute or strict, 83–91
    corporate, 89–91
    criminal, 87–89
    employer, 87–91
    general, 81–91
    manufacturer's, 86
    product, 84
    professionals and managers, 86–87

Magnetic resonance imaging (MRI scan), 44
Manganese, 182–183
Mercury, 1, 45, 74
    organic, 184–188
Methyl isocyanate, 82

Negligence, 82
Nerve conduction velocity (NCV), 57–60, 64
    aging effects, 74
    choice of nerves, 57–60, 74
    nerve temperature, 74
    use in a screening program, 73–75
Nervous system, reasons for monitoring, 40–41, 45–60
Neurophysiological testing, 55–60, 64, 73–75
Neuropsychology, 53–55, 91
    examinations, 94–147
Neurotoxicity, and cancer, 28–29
    case reports, 94–148
    delayed effects, 26–27, 29–30
    effects of low-level exposure, 20
    employee monitoring for, 64–67
    epidemiology, 15–24
    evaluation of, 40–60, 91, 94–147
    family exposure, 139–148
    forensic, 91
    prevention, 64–77
    ramifications of, 24–27
    screening program, 64–77
    symptoms of, 3–8, 45, 46–51, 64, 68
    threshold effects, 28
    treatment of, 76–77
Neurotoxicity screening program,
    applications, 65
    data analysis, 75–76
    design, 65–77
    purpose of, 65
    repeated measurement, 72–73
    statistical aspects, 66–67
Neurotoxicity Screening Survey, 46–51, 68

Organophosphates
    case reports, 99–114
    general, 2
    toxicity of, 188–193

Painting, spray, case report, 122–126
Peripheral nerve testing, 57–60. Also see
    Nerve conduction velocity

Pesticides, 2, 35
    case reports, 99–114
    in food, 19–22, 34–36
    tolerance levels, 21–22
    toxicity of, 188–193
Phorate
    case report, 99–109
    toxicity of, 192
Polychlorinated biphenyl (PCB), 42
    case report, 114–122
    toxicity of, 193–199
Positive emission tomography (PET scan), 44
Pre-exposure function, estimates of, 54–55
Pressed wood products, 176–178
Product warnings, 64
Psycho-organic syndrome, 88
Psychometric tests, 45–55
    batteries of, 52–53
    case reports, 94–148
    computerized, 53
    in a screening program, 68–73

Radiation, 200–207
Risk assessment, 27–28

Solvents, 24, 35, 45
    case reports, 94–99, 122–126

Thimet
    case report, 99–109
    toxicity of, 192
Torts, intentional, 83
Torts, fraudulent misrepresent or concealment, 88–89
Toxic torts, 81–91
Toxic waste, 24
Transformer fluid contamination, case report, 114–122
Trichloroethane, 94–99

Urea formaldehyde foam insulation,
    installation, 147–148. Also see
    Formaldehyde

Warnings
    legal aspects, 84–85
    product, neurotoxicity prevention programs, 64
Worker's compensation, 87